LIZ EARLE

THE GOOD GUT GUIDE

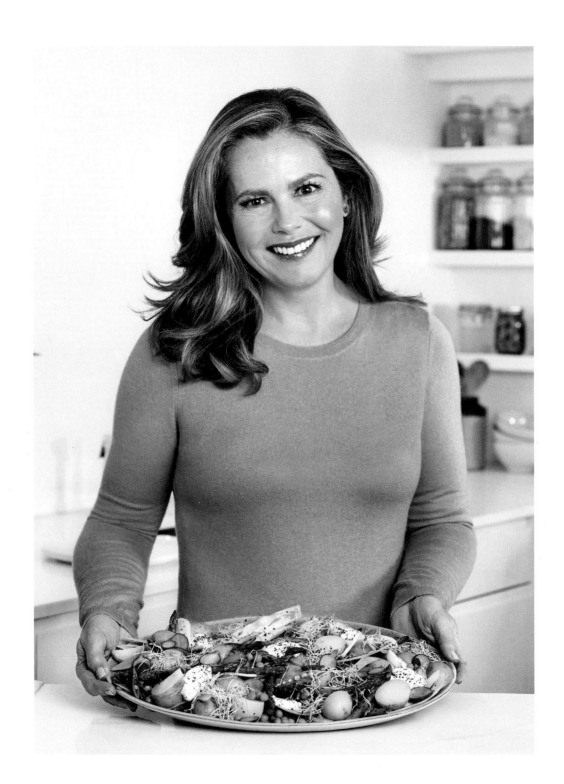

LIZ EARLE

THE GOOD GUT GUIDE

DELICIOUS RECIPES
AND A SIMPLE 6-WEEK PLAN FOR
INNER HEALTH AND OUTER BEAUTY

First published in Great Britain in 2017 by Orion Spring
an imprint of The Orion Publishing Group Ltd
Carmelite House, 50 Victoria Embankment
London EC4Y 0DZ

An Hachette UK Company

1 3 5 7 9 10 8 6 4 2

Photographer: Dan Jones
Creative Director: Helen Ewing
Project Editor: Olivia Morris
Home Economist and Food Stylist: Natalie Thomson
Props Stylist: Tamzin Ferdinando
Nutritional analysis calculated by: Fiona Hunter BSc (hons) Nutrition, Diploma Dietetics
Illustrator: Amy Louise Evans

Every effort has been made to ensure that the information in the book is accurate.
The information in this book may not be applicable in each individual case so it is advised
that professional medical advice is obtained for specific health matters and before changing
any medication or dosage. Neither the publisher nor author accepts any legal responsibility
for any personal injury or other damage or loss arising from the use of the information in
this book. In addition, if you are concerned about your diet or exercise regime and wish to
change them, you should consult a health practitioner first.

A CIP catalogue record for this book is available from the British Library.

ISBN: 978 1 4091 6416 6

Printed in Italy

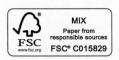

MIX
Paper from
responsible sources
FSC® C015829
FSC
www.fsc.org

www.orionbooks.co.uk

ORION
SPRING

Contents

Preface

Over the last thirty years, my research and writing have looked at how we can best improve our outer beauty and inner wellbeing. My first books from 1990 pioneered the benefits of 'good' fats and oils in our diet, and I took an early look at antioxidants with some of the first consumer guides on wellness subjects, from juicing to herbs for health, eating for better skin and so much more. Over the years, I've written a great deal on the subject of eating to look younger and leaner, feel better and live stronger. But this book digs deeper than all of these put together. I could not have written this book until now. Modern science and medicine are only just uncovering the secrets of gut health and why it has the power to totally transform the way we look and feel. Not only can I reveal here what we all *really* need to eat (and drink) to improve our health and wellbeing, I will explain how the microscopic organisms that make up so much of who we are also make the most incredible difference to how we look, how well we age and how fit we feel. It's the most significant book I have ever written.

And the stars of this story? Well, they're so small that they're invisible to the naked eye. So tiny you could place millions onto a single pin-head. Yet so mighty in strength and impact, they make all the difference in the world between being happy or sad, having good skin or bad, energy or lethargy — even life or death itself. I'm talking about the marvellous world of microbes, a complex community of beneficial bacteria that each and every one of us has within us and which makes up our very own internal 'microbiome'.

Much has been written on the subject of gut health in the last year or two. Most of it from either a scientific or medical perspective. I've enjoyed reading books from my fellow authors on this subject, but have always been left wanting to know more. Understanding the science and medical statistics is fascinating stuff, but as a working woman and mother of five, I want to know how I can put this new-found knowledge to good, practical use in everyday life. It's all very well knowing that our gut flora can keep us slim, sane and strong, but how exactly do we do this? How come some everyday foods boost our beneficial bacteria while others have the opposite effect? What are the best things to eat and drink? How do friendly flora keep our skin smooth and wrinkles at bay? Where do good microbes come from? Which ones do we need? What should we be doing for our children? For the elderly? For the sick and those desperately searching for better health?

My own personal journey to find the answers to these questions and more, for my own family and for me, has been the driving force behind this book.

More than any other, this is a book that I just *had* to publish. And I'm so grateful to my editors at Orion Spring for listening to my many impassioned pleas and allowing me the resources to research and write *The Good Gut Guide*. What I have found is so mind-blowing that it actually takes my breath away. It's no wonder that almost every area of medical science is now focusing on the gut and its magnificent, mighty microbiome. From ageing to obesity, arthritis to depression, cancer to cardiology, our microflora are firmly in charge and running the show. So I invite you now to come along with me on an incredible six-week journey to discover what lies within the deepest recesses of your being – and how a world so minutely microscopic is making the biggest difference to how we look, feel and live. I'll share with you the science, the studies, the most successful strategies and superior sources of these microbial marvels, as well as how best to collect, cultivate and protect friendly flora and beneficial bacteria with tasty and interesting recipes. I'll introduce you to a new internal landscape and share with you a whole new language of pre- and probiotics, starter cultures and fermented foods that will set you up with a formidable taskforce of new-found friends for life.

Accessible and easy to make, I've taste-tested my recipes on my own family – and love the way I now have some real control over what my family and I need to help us stay healthy and strong. I've provided nutritional advice along the way, especially for those with digestive issues, with the help of dietitian Fiona Hunter and include calorie counts per serving (where ranges are given, the smaller number of calories relates to the larger number of servings) as well as these symbols for:

V VEGETARIAN

DF DAIRY-FREE

GF GLUTEN-FREE

I hope you love following my six-week plan to better health, beauty and wellbeing. I'd love to hear how you get on, so please share your stories along the way using #goodgutguide and #gutfood to show and inspire others on the journey to wellbeing – you'll find all my contact details on page 256.

With love,

Liz x

Liz Earle MBE
Lizearlewellbeing

Introduction

The microbiome

WHAT IS A MICROBIOME?

'Microbiome' is the term most commonly used to describe the trillions of microscopic organisms living inside our gut, which are mostly bacteria but also consist of some viruses and fungi. Any environment can have a microbiome – a plant, a refrigerator, a building, even a whole city. It's basically all the living organisms that inhabit the structure in question. It may sound pretty gross to think about a load of bacteria breeding inside us, but the reality is that we all rely heavily on this mini-ecosystem to keep us healthy and strong.

These microbes, and the balance between good and bad, play an absolutely vital role in health and disease. Our bacteria are unique to each of us and they all have to get along and work together for us to stay healthy. These bacteria feed on what we eat and drink, helping not only to break down the food to create energy, but also to manufacture essential enzymes and vitamins, and to regulate our immune system. So when we eat, we're not only fuelling our own bodies, but feeding our microbes so they flourish too.

But precisely *what* we eat encourages different types of bacteria to grow. If we eat food that nourishes the good guys, our health too will be good. But if we don't look after our microbial friends, they soon desert us, leaving us more susceptible to hostile microbial foes. I'll be taking a closer look at the foods that can help – and hinder – our microscopic mates a little later in the book.

Why such a hot topic?

It's only within the past few decades, and more specifically the past couple of years, that the contents of our intestines and the way our microbiomes work have come under the spotlight when it comes to health. Previously, there wasn't thought to be a link between the foods we ate and any particular health conditions we developed – at least, not by mainstream doctors. Only 'health nuts' – myself included – kept beating the drum, saying, 'We are what we eat.' But now, countless conditions, specifically autoimmune ones, are being linked scientifically to gut health.

So what is it that's got scientists across the globe so excited about our intestines? Quite simply, microbes. We all have 100 trillion bacteria living naturally in our bodies, most of which are housed in the gastrointestinal (GI) tract. Some are also found on the surface of our skin, and later I'll share with you a few very simple skincare secrets that will change the way your skin's ecology behaves so as to make your complexion glow.

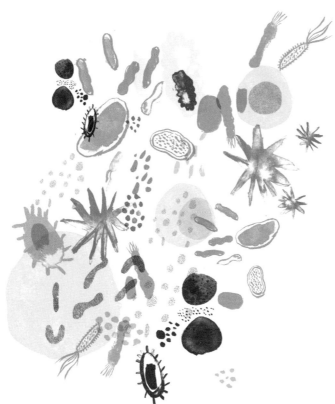

The microbiome: an array of bacteria in our internal ecosystem

What we eat affects our gut health

One of the most exciting developments is that the DNA-sequencing technology originally developed for the successful Human Genome Project is now also being used to sequence the genes of our microbes. This gives scientists a much more comprehensive understanding of the microbes inside us, how they work, what diseases they can cause, and how much we rely on them for full body health. Another exciting development has been the launch of the British Gut project in 2014 by the Department of Twin Research at King's College London.

The aim of the project was, and still is, to delve into the microbial diversity of our guts. Members of the public are encouraged to take part by sending off samples of microbes from their gut, skin and mouth, to see how these are affected by food and lifestyle choices. The project has used dietary interventions such as cheese- and yoghurt-heavy diets, dietary cleanses using only plant foods, and fasting to show how what we eat can cause a change to our gut's microbial diversity within just a few days. It has proven that although on a genetic level we humans are all 99 per cent the same, our microbiomes vary a great deal and can even affect how much weight we gain. This may be the reason why some of us have amazing success on a particular diet but others see no benefit at all. It's also why some can eat carbs until the cows come home, while others blow up like a balloon at the mere whiff of a plate of pasta. The American Gut project is a similar set-up across the ocean and one of the largest crowd-sourced research projects in the United States. As more research is conducted into gut microbes around the globe, scientists are predicting with greater accuracy than ever before which food choices and diets will work best for which of us.

How the gut works

In order to understand where and how bacteria play such an important part, let's take a look at how the digestive system works. The GI tract is effectively a long tube running from one end of our body to the other. This piece of internal plumbing starts with swallowing food, digesting it to absorb its energy and nutrients, and then excreting the waste matter at the other end of the system.

THE STOMACH

After food has passed down the throat (oesophagus) it reaches the stomach, where very few bacteria survive the potent mix of digestive juices, made up of bile, enzymes and hydrochloric acid. The pH of a normal, empty stomach is generally around 1.5–2, which is extremely acidic. This serves an important purpose, as the acid kills off invading pathogenic bacteria and viruses. The digestive juices quickly get to work breaking down the food into what's called 'chyme', a thick gloopy liquid, ready to pass on to the small intestine.

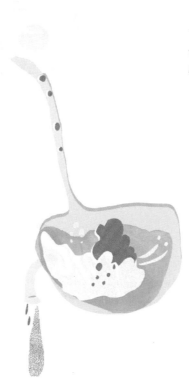

The GI tract is one long tube with our intestines in the middle

THE SMALL INTESTINE

This 20-foot-long section of our GI tract is made up of the duodenum, jejunum and ileum. It runs from our stomach to the beginning of the large intestine, and it's here that 90 per cent of the digestion and absorption of food takes place. After the chyme is emptied from the stomach into the duodenum, bile is added from the gall bladder along with digestive juices from the pancreas. These neutralise the acids from the stomach so the absorption of vitamins, minerals and nutrients can then begin.

Next, the chyme enters the jejunum, which is responsible for the absorption of most of the nutrients. Here, sugar in the form of glucose and amino acids from proteins are absorbed into the lining of the intestine, while fats are absorbed into the lymph vessels.

Lastly, the chyme reaches the ileum, which manufactures and absorbs vitamin B12 and bile salts. Any remaining undigested or unabsorbed food passes into the large intestine. In terms of bacteria, there are around 10,000 microbes per millilitre of gut at the beginning of the small intestine, increasing to 10 million at the end where the large intestine begins. That's a lot of bugs working hard in a small but important space.

THE LARGE INTESTINE

The first section of the large intestine is the caecum, a hothouse of microbial activity. This roundish chamber is home to *trillions* of individual microbes, which thrive on the partially digested leftover food – mainly the fibrous parts of plants that are still intact, which the bacteria here get to feed on.

From the caecum, food then enters the colon, which is the largest part of our large intestine. There are as many as 500 species of bacteria living in our colon. Many of these are particularly adept at breaking down the tough cellulose and pectin (a gel-like substance) found in plant cells and fibres, and turning them into simple sugars, which are then fermented to create short-chain fatty acids (SCFAs) that can be absorbed. These substances are thought to make up 10 per cent of our calorie intake.

The health of our colon depends almost entirely on these SCFAs, unlike other cells in our body, which require glucose for energy. This is one reason why plant-based dietary fibre is so vital for good gut health – it's not all about roughage, but also about feeding our beneficial bacteria with this prebiotic fibre. So we need to eat plenty of plants.

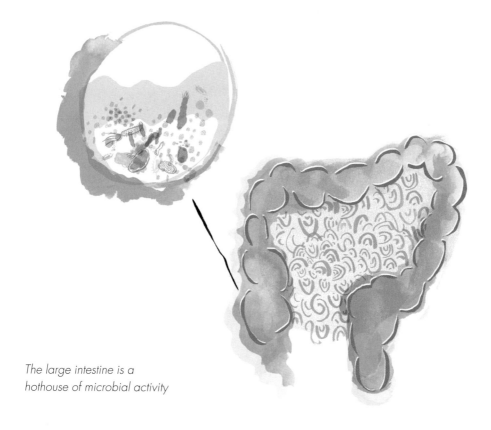

The large intestine is a hothouse of microbial activity

THE APPENDIX

Once thought to be a prehistoric part of our digestive system, the appendix turns out to be rather useful after all, as it's a storehouse of good bacteria. In previous centuries, when it was far more likely we'd become ill with dysentery or other water-borne diseases, after the microbes had been flushed out of the system our appendix would repopulate the gut with good bacteria – a topping-up mechanism. The appendix is actually part of our lymphatic system, strategically located at the point where our small and large intestines meet, and it provides a 'trap' where bad bugs can be caught and destroyed. The once overlooked appendix is now being linked to providing protection from gastrointestinal infections, some autoimmune diseases, cancer of the blood and heart attacks – all thanks to its stockpile of microbes. Once it is removed, we lose part of our immune system, so it's an important decision to discuss with medics, bearing in mind that such a course should be taken only when in dire need (its removal can save your life, though, in the case of peritonitis).

But if you have had your appendix removed, don't panic, just be aware. Specialists such as the natural health doctor David Williams recommend a regular supply of probiotics (see page 52) as a form of cheap insurance: 'Because you no longer have the reservoir of good bacteria, daily replenishment is a good idea.'

Tummy troubles

Now that we understand a little about the basics of how our digestive system works, let's look at some of the best ways to spot poor gut health. Each of us has our own unique microbiome, and it's when it gets out of balance, perhaps slowly over time through poor eating habits, or rapidly from a course of high-strength antibiotics or a virus, that 'dysbiosis' occurs. Dysbiosis, or a dysfunctional microbiome, means that pathogenic strains of bacteria or viruses can take hold and lead to ill-health and susceptibility to certain conditions, such as cancer, heart disease, obesity and autoimmune diseases. It's this dysfunctional mix of microbes that is at the root of so many of today's modern illnesses, which we'll come to in more detail later.

Bad-gut giveaways

These are some of the more obvious signs that our gut health has gone awry:

- **Bloating and constipation**
  Constipation may be the most obvious cause of bloating and can lead to stools (faeces) remaining in the intestines, causing the stomach area to feel hard, as well as pain, discomfort and windy gas. The causes of constipation include too little fibre, not drinking enough water, lack of physical exercise, and the side effects of medication and stress. Bloating can also occur as a result of dehydration because lack of water plus electrolyte (body salts) imbalances can

halt digestion. 'This is because when your body attempts to counterbalance the effects of being dehydrated, it holds on to excess water which leads to bloating,' says Dr Ayesha Akbar, consultant gastroenterologist at St Mark's Hospital, London.

- **Indigestion and acid reflux**
All foods need specific enzymes to break them down, and sometimes when we've ingested too many different foods in a meal it can be difficult for our stomach to deal with them all at once. Acid reflux can often be caused by a lack of, rather than too much, stomach acid. We'll cover this in more detail in Week Two.

- **Recurrent pain or cramping**
If you get pains within 20 to 30 minutes of eating anything with gluten in it, this might mean you have an intolerance to gluten (see page 16) or may even have coeliac disease (there are many other symptoms, such as itchy skin rashes, fatigue, joint pain and even irritability, so it can be hard to diagnose – visit coeliac.org.uk for more on this). In the last few decades, gluten appears to have become difficult for many of us to process, perhaps because of the way the strains of modern wheat are commercially bred and farmed. Whatever the reason, gluten can act a bit like glue, gumming up our intestines to a lesser or greater extent (depending on our personal sensitivity) and causing inflammation. From cereals and toast for breakfast, to morning biscuits, a lunchtime sandwich, a teatime cake, then pasta, pizza

or pastry for supper, the chances are all of us probably eat too much gluten during an average day. If you experience pain in your small intestine, this may be a sign all is not well and you need to cut back on gluten and pay your gut a little more care and attention.

- **Bad breath**
The reason for bad breath isn't always poor oral hygiene. If you're not properly digesting food and it's putrefying in your intestines, it can produce noxious gasses that travel back up your windpipe and result in bad breath. We also have beneficial microbes in our saliva, which need protecting and preserving to help here (and not be destroyed with chemical mouthwashes).

- **Unusual stool movements**
Ideally, you would have a small soft bowel movement after each meal, but very few people experience that, apart from babies! Going to the loo once a day is considered normal, but it ought not to be difficult. Being constipated is one cause of infrequent bowel movements. If you're not passing a soft stool at least once a day, you're considered to have constipation. Any straining means the stool is either too large or too hard, both of which indicate the faeces have been sitting inside your colon for too long. At the other end of the scale, very loose stools can lead to dehydration and may also be a symptom of a food intolerance or 'leaky gut' (see page 18). If you have bleeding from your back passage, always get this checked by your doctor.

What's up, gut?

The aforementioned are unpleasant enough, but they can sometimes be symptoms of more serious underlying conditions, including a whole host of seemingly unrelated health complaints, from skin rashes to other autoimmune issues such as multiple sclerosis (MS) and diabetes.

Irritable bowel syndrome (IBS)

For some, the symptoms I've described are all too common and they may be characteristic of the group estimated at 10–20 per cent of the UK population that is affected by IBS. One in every five of us in the Western world now has the condition and, oddly, twice as many women as men seem to be affected. The precise causes are still relatively unknown, but the condition is characterised by constipation and/or diarrhoea, bloating and abdominal pain. Although the bowel may show no signs of inflammation, this is not necessarily to say that the digestive system is working normally. 'Our intestines are made up of a complicated system of nerves, and IBS is caused by a loss of coordination within this system and the way the bowel works. Therefore, sufferers of IBS have nothing structurally wrong but something functionally wrong,' says Dr Akbar.

Some now believe IBS might be triggered by an infection or a dose of food poisoning, after which the intestine never quite recovers. Alanna Collen, science writer and author of *10% Human: How Your Body's Microbes Hold the Key to Health and Happiness*, points out that those who get traveller's diarrhoea are around seven times more likely to develop IBS later in life. She also says antibiotics could be another cause although, confusingly, in some people they actually help alleviate symptoms. This all makes it very hard to identify one single cause of IBS.

Inflammatory bowel disease (IBD)

IBD is a chronic inflammatory disorder of the gut, and includes Crohn's disease, ulcerative colitis and small intestinal bowel overgrowth (SIBO). The main symptoms here include diarrhoea, blood in the stools, tummy pains and weight loss. 'In addition, IBD can lead to bloating. A major cause of bloating is gas, which can become trapped in the bowels or is expelled as wind. IBD sufferers may also experience bloating if they have scar tissue (adhesions) as a result of previous surgery,' says Dr Akbar.

Coeliac disease

This autoimmune disease has symptoms that are triggered by a protein found in gluten, which is present in grains such as barley, rye and wheat. Gluten damages the lining of the small intestine and, in some cases, other parts of the body. Commonly recognised symptoms include constipation, diarrhoea and excessive wind, gastrointestinal symptoms such as nausea and vomiting, and discomfort from bloating and cramping. Coeliac disease can lead to headaches and fatigue, weight loss, depression and deficiencies in folic acid, iron or vitamin B12. It can also cause skin rashes, osteoporosis, pain in the bones and joints, neurological conditions including poor muscle coordination as well as numbness and tingling in the hands and feet. It's a serious disorder – and not to be confused with a mild gluten sensitivity.

Non-coeliac gluten sensitivity (NCGS)

For some, it may not be gluten that's causing the problem, but another type of protein in wheat called amylase-trypsin inhibitors (ATIs). Although ATIs account for only 4 per cent of wheat proteins, they have been found to trigger powerful immune reactions that can spread from the intestines to other parts of the body. It's also thought ATIs might worsen the symptoms of rheumatoid arthritis, MS, asthma, lupus and IBD. Because of this new information, NCGS may end up needing a new name if gluten isn't the main trigger cause after all. This research is cutting-edge – watch this space!

Weight gain

Incredibly, being overweight could also be caused in part by the mix of microbes in our intestine. In fact, gut health and its influence on obesity is now one of the fastest-growing areas of study in the scientific community, and for good reason: worldwide, one in three adults is overweight and one in ten is classed as obese. Being obese is linked to many other conditions such as heart disease, cancer, depression, anxiety and diabetes. But rather than obesity being down to our genetics, as was previously thought, it turns out to have far more to do with gut microbes than with DNA. Only a tiny 32 genes out of our 21,000 have been found to play a role in weight gain. Recent research confirms that it's not necessarily the number of calories we consume that causes weight gain, but what the bugs in our tummy actually do with that food.

This discovery may be largely down to which particular bugs are living in our microbial communities. As you'll read later on in this book, there's a group of bacteria called *Akkermansia* that's often missing in the guts of those who are overweight, yet makes up around 4 per cent of the overall microbiome of those who are within a healthy weight range. It's not known how or why *Akkermansia* bacteria either die off or are absent, but scientists have found that a high-fibre diet can boost their numbers back up. Indeed, they have known gut bacteria can affect our weight ever since doctors started performing faecal-matter transplants, where microbes are collected from the colons of healthy people and put into those with severe infectious diseases who have not responded to antibiotics. A kind of pass-the-poo treatment.

In addition to bacteria such as *Akkermansia*, another group of bugs known as firmicutes has also been shown to influence weight gain. A test on 977 volunteers found that those with higher levels of firmicutes called *Christensenella* were more likely to be leaner than those with low levels. If you're looking to lose weight, bugs such as *Akkermansia* and firmicutes could become your new best flora friends.

Allergies

Back in the 1930s it was rare for children to have asthma; perhaps only one child in every school had it. But by the 1980s, around one in every classroom had the condition. A similar thing happened with peanut allergies, which trebled in the 1990s and then doubled over the next five years. Allergies are now being strongly linked to poor bacterial diversity, especially in those who were not exposed to enough microbes at an early age. The number of times antibiotics are administered to a child, especially those under the age of two, can also increase the likelihood of having allergies later in life.

Food allergies, sensitivities or intolerances can lead to stomach bloating. The two most common food groups that trigger this are dairy products and foods containing gluten, alongside nuts, peanuts (a legume, not technically a nut), eggs and soya.

Autoimmune diseases

The term 'autoimmune disease' is used to describe a situation where our own immune system inadvertently attacks our body because it gets confused and thinks harmless substances, such as pollen, food particles or dust, are harmful. How an autoimmune disease manifests itself varies dramatically from person to person, from a simple but annoying skin breakout to MS or chronic fatigue – or a combination of many. Some of the better-known autoimmune disorders are eczema, psoriasis, dermatitis, IBS, IBD, Crohn's disease, lupus, MS and type 2 diabetes. Under normal conditions, our immune system prevents invading infectious diseases from taking hold. And as 60–70 per cent of our immune cells are actually found in our gut, you can see why good gut health can significantly help guard against autoimmune diseases.

Mental wellbeing

This is perhaps the most unexpected and fascinating of all areas of gut-health research – the fact that the microbes in our gut affect our mental health, our moods and emotions, and may be implicated in depression, violent behaviour and even self-harm. Psychologists of the past used to view all mental disorders as purely brain-based, but there is growing evidence to suggest many mind-centred conditions actually begin in the gut – you may have heard the gut referred to as the 'second brain'. Many of the trillions of cells in our gut are in fact neurotransmitters, the so-called brain chemicals we used to think were only produced by the brain. This explains 'gut feelings', because our intestines are acting as a barometer for how we feel and transmitting the 'readings' up to our brain. From low moods through to full-blown schizophrenia, autism, dementia and Parkinson's, an unbalanced microbiome is now often implicated. We'll come to mental wellbeing in much more detail a little later, as well as take a look at how stress affects the gut in Week Five, when we'll investigate in more depth the fascinating gut–brain connection.

SO WHAT IS A LEAKY GUT?

In essence, a leaky gut is one that is more permeable and leaking more than it should. The gut is designed to allow some molecules through – that's how we absorb nutrients from our food. But if the lining becomes inflamed due to too much junk food, a sensitivity to gluten or an over-reliance on prescription drugs, the microbe balance can be thrown off and lead to damage within the gut lining. All the little finger-like projections (the villi) that stick up like the shagpile on a carpet and coat our insides can get worn down and develop gaps between them, allowing larger particles, such as undigested food, through to the bloodstream. When this happens, it alerts immune HQ that an unwanted 'invader' has entered our system, which in turn sets off an inflammatory reaction to surround those unwelcome particles and neutralise them. Leaky gut is now thought to be responsible for the rapid rise in autoimmune conditions throughout the Western world.

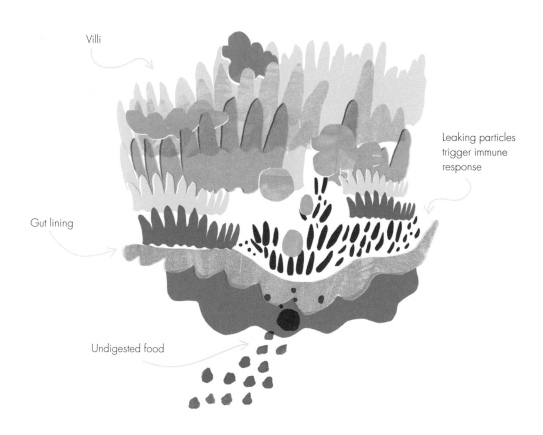

Villi

Leaking particles trigger immune response

Gut lining

Undigested food

Poor skin health

The outer state of our skin is one of the simplest barometers for assessing inner gut health. How we look on the outside is a pretty accurate reflection of what's happening on the inside – and one of the best ways to get great skin is via better gut health. Our skin is the most important line of defence against the outside world. It's a carefully constructed barrier that's highly efficient at keeping microscopic bugs, bacteria and viruses from invading our bodies. It's a complete beauty myth that products applied to the surface of the skin can somehow slip through it and enter the bloodstream – the particle sizes used in beauty products are vastly bigger than the microbes our skin is so cleverly designed to keep out. But did you know that the skin is an essential part of our immune system and profoundly reliant on certain colonies of bacteria on its surface to keep it healthy? If these get damaged, we lay ourselves open to invasions from a variety of unwanted bugs.

Around one thousand different types of bacteria live on our skin, and we have about a trillion inhabiting our epidermis (outer skin) and hair follicles at any given moment. These are typically non-harmful and can even do us good by combating the bad bugs that lead to disease.

Interestingly, these beneficial microbes on the skin's surface have an important role to play in our inner health too. Recent studies show there is a clear gut–brain–skin relationship and that our inner microbes affect our outer skin. Science is now revealing how our skin can 'think' and communicate with our brain. Known as the NICE (neuro-immuno-cutaneous-endocrine) network, this consists of our nervous system, immune system, plus our skin and hormone systems. These are linked together by microbial messengers that 'talk' to each other, passing on information and instructions. When one part communicates, the others listen and respond.

I have always held that the secret of clear, smooth, glowing skin has as much to do with what we eat as it has to do with skincare, but it's interesting to learn that it's how well we look after our inner gut health, specifically with probiotics and fermented foods, that gives us more radiant-looking skin. Modern medicine is being turned on its head: instead of using *antibiotics* to treat skin disorders, many medics are now turning to *probiotics* for those hard-to-treat dermatological problems.

Simple maths: better gut = better health

Entire textbooks have been written on all of the above, so what you have just read is only a short overview, but I hope you can already see that there are so many valid, important reasons why we need to get to grips with what's going on in our gut and make the most of our microbes. A better gut means better health. It really is that simple. And it works at every level of the body, as friendly microbes affect not only the digestion of our food but also our brain health, mood, emotions, energy levels, ageing, weight loss and so much more. Understanding this can give us the blueprint for a longer, happier, healthier life – which is why I believe *The Good Gut Guide* to be such a fundamentally important book for us all. So let's get ready to begin our first week, which starts with inner cleansing and flushing out the bad bugs before we can properly repopulate with more of the good guys.

PART ONE: SIX-WEEK PLAN

WEEK ONE:
Detox

Do you need to detox? Well, if you've ever taken a course of antibiotics the chances are your microbiome could do with a boost, and even if you're not someone with a digestive disorder (such as IBS, reflux or leaky gut) my view is that cleansing the system before repopulating with beneficial microflora gives us the best chance for optimum health and long-term wellbeing. Given the enormous amount of processed foods and sugary drinks available to us these days, not to mention the array of prescription drugs, especially antibiotics, that have been dished out so readily, it's no wonder our insides are struggling to cope and could do with a clean-out.

Science is proving that if we take care of our gut by giving it the best possible foods and probiotics, and make time to relax and enjoy our meals, we can create better health and wellbeing from the inside out. In Week One, my focus is on clearing away unwanted waste matter from the gut, including possible yeast overgrowths, bad bacteria and even parasites that can block better gut health.

① Resting our gut

It's really important to allow our body, and therefore our gut, to rest from time to time. Far from being a new-fangled trend, missing meals (or fasting) for one day or even a week, has been practised for thousands of years. And the reason that having a break from food can be beneficial is because digestion takes up an awful lot of energy and diverts attention away from healing and repairing. In fact, digestion often takes precedence over all other processes – unless we're in extreme fight-or-flight mode, in which case it shuts down temporarily until the threat has passed. So if there's essential maintenance work needed, such as repairing an internal organ or the skin, this will be put on hold while digestion is under way. That's because our body only has limited resources and energy, and has to prioritise.

Another good reason to give our gut a rest can be found in recent studies looking at one of the main groups of bacteria – known as Firmicutes – found in greater numbers in those who are overweight. These microbes extract more calories, especially fat, from food and they increase in number when given a high-calorie diet yet dwindle when deprived of food, say on a 24-hour fast. This is perhaps one of the reasons why intermittent fasting works so well both for weight loss and for regulating blood sugar levels.

Cutting our food intake became popular with the 5:2 diet, but there's an even easier way to do intermittent fasting, and that's simply by leaving a clear 12-hour gap between your last meal of the day and your first one the next day. A small adjustment to our mealtimes can make a big difference to our gut health, especially in relation to weight gain if this change leads to a reduction in food-fattening Firmicutes.

TRY A SHORT FAST

- At the beginning of this detox week consider having a whole day of not eating anything solid, to give your body a chance to properly rest and start the healing process. Juices, broths, herbal teas and plenty of water are all fine (and recommended).

- Rest your gut overnight, calculating a clear 12-hour window when nothing is eaten – for example, finishing your last meal of the day by 8 p.m. and beginning breakfast at 8 a.m., or later.

② Foods to eliminate

ADDED SUGARS AND SWEETENERS: It's been shown that artificial sweeteners can alter the make-up of our microbiome, causing imbalance and, over time, even leading to weight gain or type 2 diabetes.

So, during this week, and for as long as possible, try cutting out all sources of unnatural sweeteners. You can do this by eliminating processed, pre-packaged sugary foods and drinks as they often contain them. This includes, but is not limited to, sweets, cakes, pastries, fizzy drinks, flavoured waters, chewing gum and some yoghurts – do read the labels to check for hidden sweeteners such as acesulfame K, aspartame, saccharin and sucralose.

Other sugars worth cutting down on – or out completely for these six weeks – are the calorific sugars that originate from natural sugar but are so processed that they can be damaging in large volumes. Read the food labels and try to avoid the following: dextrose, glucose syrup, crystalline fructose, high-fructose corn syrup, fruit juice concentrates, maltodextrin and trehalose. Some people also have problems with sugar alcohols such as xylitol and maltitol (all those ending in -tol), as although they can come from natural sources they often cause digestive complaints, such as having a laxative effect, especially for those who are sensitive to FODMAP foods (see page 42).

DRIED FRUITS: Even though fructose (and some other sugars) come from fruits, and fruit is not bad *per se*, the dried varieties are the health-store equivalent of chocolate buttons – they send our blood sugar rocketing and will feed any overgrowth of candida (an internal yeast) you may have. By all means introduce a few dried apricots, dates and prunes later on in the schedule, but it's best to avoid them for the first few weeks as you detox and cleanse.

TOP TIP: If you're craving sweetness, try a teaspoon of raw (unprocessed) honey in a cup of herbal tea, or use stevia – a naturally sweet plant – to sweeten home baking.

GLUTEN: Social media has gone crazy for gluten-free, and while it's true that only a few of us – that is, those with coeliac disease – have a real need to cut it out completely, there's growing evidence that more of us are becoming sensitive to it, hence the rise in the condition known as non-coeliac gluten sensitivity (as discussed on page 16). Much of this problem may lie in the way modern strains of wheat are bred and milled into flour. Animal studies show that glyphosate, the pesticide increasingly used to grow genetically modified (GM) wheat, negatively affects gut health. Some researchers have speculated that the rise in glyphosate residues (especially in bread) could be contributing to the rise in modern diseases worldwide – not only for coeliac disease and gluten intolerance, but also potentially for ADHD (attention deficit hyperactivity disorder), autism, Alzheimer's disease, infertility and cancer.

One way to avoid glyphosate residues is to buy organic bread and bake with organic flours. If you are sensitive to ordinary bread you may find sourdough a better option, as it's fermented and easier to digest.

ALCOHOL: While the odd glass of red wine could actually be beneficial for our health, for these six weeks you'll want to give your gut the best chance of healing. Cutting out alcohol which, along with the sugar and sweeteners, feeds bacterial overgrowths, is a good way to maximise the effectiveness of the plan. And anyway, I expect you'll soon be so taken with my Kvass (page 238) and Kombucha (page 104) concoctions that these gut-healing drinks will become your new tipples of choice!

ANTIBIOTICS

While it's sometimes essential to take a course of antibiotics if you have a serious bacterial infection (including dental infections), or you've picked up a bug abroad, for example, it's best to avoid them where at all possible, as too much reliance on these pharmaceutical drugs disrupts our microbiome. This is because they act to kill off so many bacteria, not just the specific ones causing you to be unwell. The result is that your microbiome is weakened, and the wrong sorts of bacteria can start to take hold when this state prevails.

It's essential to take a course of probiotics at the same time as antibiotics, to mitigate as much of the damage as possible. Then follow up with a potent probiotic repopulating regime (see Week Three). What's more, the overuse of antibiotics – and anything designed to kill bacteria, such as antibacterial handwashes – is leading to worldwide antibiotic resistance. This is a serious problem because within a few decades we're likely to have run out of effective antibiotics – yet another reason to take them only if you absolutely have to, so that when you do need them, they work.

③ A clean sweep

During this detox week you might like to try a systematic approach to cleansing your lower intestine. You'll no doubt have heard of colonic irrigation as a method of detoxing, for removing not only parasites, bad bacteria and viruses but also food that may have become impacted over time and is putrefying – nice! While this therapy can be beneficial when carried out by a trained practitioner, there are other less invasive and cheaper ways to cleanse your lower intestine, such as with drinks you can prepare easily at home as part of this first week of inner cleansing.

The bentonite clay cleanse

This is a classic and highly effective intestinal cleanse that has been practised by European naturopaths and some doctors for decades. Popular on the continent, it's a way of helping the gut clear out some of the bad stuff with a gentle clay cleanse, and without needing to fast. Bentonite clay (also known as Montmorillonite clay) is made of volcanic ash, which is rich in iron, magnesium and silicon. It isn't absorbed by the body when ingested, but passes through the system mopping up waste matter, pesticide residues and heavy metals along the way – basically acting as a highly absorbent sponge to clean out our insides.

A clay cleanse can help remove unwanted waste matter from our GI tract as well as reducing internal inflammation, thanks to its slight laxative effect.

- Before taking bentonite clay, make sure it's grey or cream in colour, not bright white as that may mean it's gone off. It should be odourless and tasteless.

WHO WILL BENEFIT?

If, after reading through the first few pages of this book, you're feeling as though your gut could do with a thorough reboot, this kind of internal cleanse could help set you on the right path. Especially if you have taken antibiotics in the past, or if you're aware that your diet or lifestyle has not been as healthy as it might have been in years gone by. You may also like to read on to the Ages and Stages section in Week Two (pages 37–42) to see if your medical history could alert you to a greater need for a clay cleanse.

- Mix one rounded teaspoon of bentonite clay powder in a large glass of plain still water (at least 230ml) using a plastic spoon or wooden-spoon handle, as the clay is magnetic and will absorb ions from a metal one (it's this magnetic action that helps draw the toxins – the waste matter – to it).

- Stir briskly, then leave for at least 30 minutes to allow the clay to absorb some of the water.

- Before drinking, stir it up again so the clay is dispersed throughout the water.

- Drink another glass of still water immediately afterwards.

- Continue drinking plenty of water throughout the day, as you want the clay to flush through and not make you constipated.

- Do consult your doctor if you are taking any prescription medications before using, as the clay can also remove drug residues.

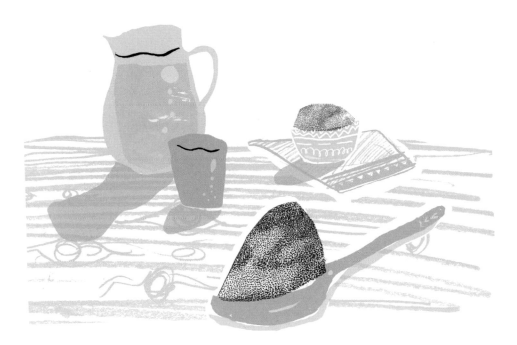

If you're starting out, each morning take the clay on an empty stomach, and then wait at least 30 minutes before eating. The clay can have a laxative effect, so be aware! Detox symptoms can include nausea, fatigue, aches and pains, a sore throat, cold sores, rashes, difficulty sleeping and flu-like symptoms. These can all indicate waste matter being drawn out of the system and into your body before excretion, so could be expected.

A MILDER METHOD: THE PSYLLIUM CLEANSE

For a less potent form of internal cleansing, try using psyllium husks or seeds. This is a milder alternative that suits those who don't fancy the more powerful clay cleanse. If you're on medication, do consult your GP and always leave a gap of two hours after taking any medicine before using psyllium (in case it removes your medication from your system before it has a chance to work).

From the Mediterranean plantain, a member of the banana family, psyllium is a form of fibre, made from the husks of the plant seeds. It comes in powdered or capsule form from most natural health stores. Its high fibre content means it absorbs a lot of water, so you must also drink much more water than usual to prevent dehydration. Psyllium husk acts as a gentle laxative and helps soothe areas of the gut that might be inflamed, which is why it's often used to treat stomach ulcers and haemorrhoids. It's also a prebiotic, meaning it feeds your good bugs (more on those in Week Five). When buying psyllium husk, look for those labelled gluten- and sugar-free and with no artificial colours, flavours or fillers.

MAKE IT YOURSELF

- Put a tablespoon of the powder into around 150ml of water, diluted juice or milk, then stir and drink immediately. Start with one serving a day and gradually work up to three. Make sure you increase your water intake, to avoid constipation.

- Avoid taking this if you have difficulty swallowing or have had narrowing of the oesophagus, or any bowel obstructions or spasms.

④ Banish bad bugs

As well as detoxing our gut to make way for a better balance of beneficial bacteria, it's worth taking a look at whether you might also benefit from trying one of the herbal detoxifiers. These are especially useful when tackling poor gut health caused by an overgrowth of bad bacteria, or if you have ever been diagnosed with any kind of severe food poisoning, *Helicobacter pylori* or parasitic infestation. Fortunately, the natural world can be relied upon to provide us with so many healing spices, herbs and other plants, many of which promote good gut health. If you know you've had an intestinal disorder, a parasitic or other bad bug such as giardia, or malaria, toxoplasmosis or worms, these are some of your natural best friends. Even the common threadworm can be deterred with a mix of pumpkin seeds and garlic (see page 33). Always check the packet instructions and seek guidance from a licensed herbal practitioner or functional medical doctor before ingesting a new herb.

Your natural medicine chest

OREGANO OIL

The dried version of the herb is a store-cupboard staple in kitchens across the UK, but this powerful plant also acts as a natural and powerful antibiotic. It's been found to fight off numerous bad bacteria, including *E. coli*, often the cause of food poisoning – so pack some next time you go abroad. Its potency is thanks to two compounds: carvacrol and thymol, both of which have antibacterial and antifungal properties.

When to take: After any kind of food poisoning, current or historic.

How to take it: You can buy oregano either in capsule form to swallow with food, or as a liquid to dilute in vegetable oil, milk or water. Taking it before eating will produce more potent results, but if you have a sensitive stomach you might want to take it after a meal. Start slowly – half the recommended dosage – and see how your body feels before increasing it.

A SAFETY NOTE: **Because of its potency, only take for a couple of weeks maximum before having a break. If you are pregnant, dried oregano (used in cooking) is fine, but the oil should be used with caution and only if prescribed by a qualified herbal practitioner.**

BERBERINE

Known as a 'natural alkaloid', this yellow compound is found in various plants including barberry and goldenseal. Taken at a low dose it is anti-inflammatory and reduces insulin resistance (see page 41). Famed for its antibacterial action, berberine has been used in traditional Chinese and Ayurvedic medicine for thousands of years. The compound has been found to alleviate gastroenteritis, diarrhoea, SIBO (see page 15) and other digestive diseases.

When to take: If you have any of these disorders, either current or historic.

How to take it: Take 500mg in capsule form 3 times a day with meals. It's best spread across the day as you need a regular intake to get maximum benefits – plus, a large dose all in one go could cause a stomach upset.

GRAPEFRUIT SEED EXTRACT

As the name suggests, this antimicrobial superstar comes from the seeds of the grapefruit, crushed along with the pulp and pith. The main compounds in the seeds – polyphenols known as limonoids and naringenin – are believed to help destroy infectious invaders. Best known for its antibacterial, antiviral and antifungal properties, it can be used to fight common health concerns, from urinary tract infections to digestive disturbances, and to kill numerous infectious microbes.

When to take: If you have had any kind of urinary tract infection, thrush (candida) or cystitis.

How to take it: A typical dose for the liquid extract is 10–12 drops in a glass of water, 1–3 times a day. Of the capsule form, take no more than 200mg, 1–3 times daily. If you're taking it for more than three consecutive days, Dr Josh Axe (a leading American nutritionist, not a medical doctor) recommends taking a probiotic (see pages 52–55) first, as too much of the extract can kill off good bacteria over the long term.

A SAFETY NOTE: Grapefruit seed extract may have been unscrupulously mixed with powerful preservatives. Avoid supplements containing benzethonium chloride or triclosan. Look for one containing just the pure grapefruit seed extract and vegetable glycerine.

OLIVE LEAF EXTRACT

This extract comes from the dried leaves of the olive tree, which are now being given almost as much attention for their healthful properties as the oil-rich olives themselves.

The olive leaf is rich in bioactive compounds that offer antioxidant benefits, and has been used for medicinal purposes since ancient Egyptian times. According to a 2003 study, olive leaves are a powerful antimicrobial with the ability to fight infections and kill bacteria and fungi, including those causing infections of the skin, hair and nails, *Candida albicans* (thrush), and *E. coli* found in the lower intestine.

When to take: A powerful antioxidant, this extract gives useful gut support and is a good choice if you are not looking to combat a more specific gut infestation.

How to take it: Steep a tablespoonful of the dried leaves in hot water for 10 minutes to make a tea. You can also buy capsules of the extract, for which follow the guidelines on the bottle. Please be aware that olive leaf extract has been known to cause dizziness in those with low blood pressure or who are taking a blood thinner.

WORMWOOD

Also known as mugwort or by its Latin name *Artemisia absinthium*, wormwood is a woody shrub with a bitter taste, used as a flavouring for vermouth. It's a powerful antifungal, antimicrobial herb and has been used for various digestive problems such as upset stomach, gall bladder disease and intestinal spasms. It continues to be used in Eastern Europe as a digestive aid and indigestion remedy.

When to take: When treating the conditions just listed. But be aware wormwood comes with a clear health warning (see safety note opposite). It is especially useful for those travelling to foreign climes where there's a possibility of picking up dangerous parasites, bugs and pathogens. It's used for expelling intestinal worms (both visible and microscopic).

How to take it: Steep half a teaspoon of the dried leaves in boiling water for 10–15 minutes. Consume this before a heavy meal as an aid to digestion. For worms or parasites, take either capsules or tincture of wormwood as directed on the packet or bottle. For gall bladder complaints, Dr Josh Axe recommends taking it in small doses for a maximum of four weeks. Dr Ann Louise Gittleman (another top American natural health practitioner) suggests drinking two cups of wormwood tea a day during your cleanse.

A SAFETY NOTE: Wormwood contains thujone and is not suitable if you have epilepsy or kidney disease or are allergic to plants in the *Asteraceae* (also called *Compositae*) family. Especially don't take it when pregnant or breastfeeding.

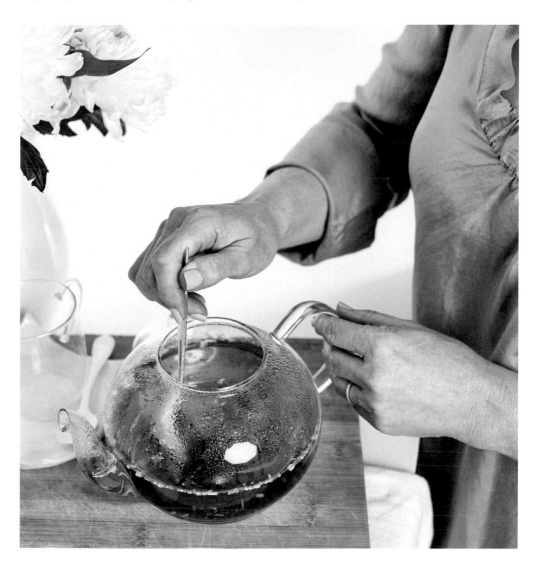

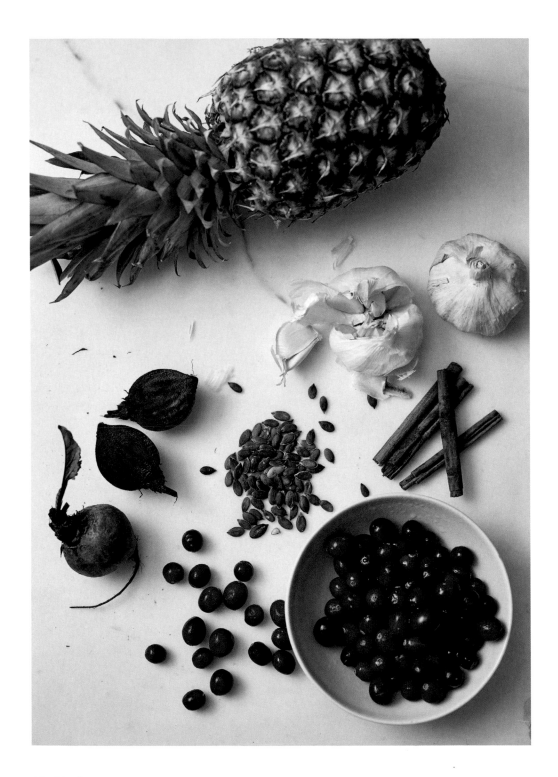

⑤ Gut food friends

Some of the best natural gut-healing ingredients can be found in the aisles of our supermarket or natural health store. This week, and throughout the plan, be sure to load up on the following:

CRANBERRIES: Fresh cranberries are packed with phenolic compounds, which help prevent bacterial overgrowth in the body. I like to sprinkle the fresh berries over a tray of oiled root vegetables, then roast for 30–40 minutes. Mixing with roasted veggies, especially if they include a few garlic bulbs, helps balance out the tartness of the berries. Or you can add them to salads or blend into coconut milk or smoothies.

PUMPKIN SEEDS: Potent internal healers, these dark-green seeds are a nutritional powerhouse containing plant protein, antioxidants called phytosterols, and a range of minerals including copper, magnesium and zinc. The large amount of zinc they contain makes them a helpful anti-parasitic, reputed to kill off intestinal parasites from harmful microbes to worms.

GARLIC: Garlic contains the natural sulphur compound allicin, which gets to work killing parasites and the bad bugs in our GI tract after about two hours of eating it. Raw or 'aged' garlic is the best. You can also take garlic capsules or tablets. Garlic is powerfully antibacterial and I always take a couple of high-strength capsules at the first sign of an infection, reducing the risk of having to resort to antibiotics. High-strength garlic supplements, combined with a tablespoonful of crushed pumpkin seeds, are an effective natural remedy for intestinal threadworms (reduce the amount for children — the smaller the child, the less required).

PINEAPPLE: This is also a good digestive fruit thanks to its enzyme bromelain, mostly found in the stalk, which is useful for breaking down proteins. It also enhances the effects of our body's own digestive enzymes trypsin and pepsin, aiding the smooth digestion of fatty foods.

BEETROOT: Beetroot is a potent blood booster and re-energiser, as well as a good support for overall liver health, which in turn supports our digestion. Try eating a daily portion during this detox week. But if eating beets every day doesn't appeal, you can juice it and add other vegetables and fruit, or try making thin beetroot crisps by finely slicing and roasting in a hot oven with a drizzle of olive oil.

CINNAMON: The spice has been used for thousands of years and has been found to fight off some pathogenic microbes. As a warming medicinal spice, cinnamon offers antioxidant, anti-inflammatory and antimicrobial properties. Try sprinkling it over cut-up root vegetables before you roast them, or add a teaspoonful to smoothies, yoghurt, milk kefir and nut milks to naturally sweeten. Also good sprinkled onto hot drinks.

GOOD-GUT CHECKLIST

1. **Cleanse your system**
Consider a gut cleanse with either bentonite clay or psyllium husk, to remove waste matter and any build-up of bad bacteria from your intestines.

2. **Try antimicrobial and anti-parasitic herbs**
Consider using bitter herbs such as oregano or wormwood, or grapefruit seed extract, to kill off any overgrowths of bad bacteria in your gut. Always read the labels and follow the directions carefully. It's often advised to seek advice from a naturopath or medical herbalist, who may prescribe you higher doses than is normally recommended on the bottles. If you do take these intestinal cleansers, use only for a week or two maximum as their effects can be powerful. As the bad bugs die off, you may experience unpleasant symptoms. This course of action is most often for those with diagnosed digestive and gut issues.

3. **Try intermittent fasting**
Something we can all benefit from. Fasting for a minimum of 12 hours while drinking plenty of water, herbal teas and fermented drinks can give your gut a rest while promoting more enzymatic activity. Consider a 24-hour fast (with plenty of fluids) on a quiet day at home this week.

4. **Love your larder**
Stock up on good-gut foods. Make sure you eat from the list of naturally gut-healing foods (see page 33) this week.

5. **Cut out known gut irritants**
What we don't eat is as important as what we do. Gluten, plus refined carbs in the form of pastries, pizzas, cakes and biscuits, are off the menu. If you have a sweet craving turn to page 238 for my Raspberry Kvass recipe – this drink will helpfully quash your sugar cravings. Give up the fizzy drinks too – unless it's the fabulous fizz from coconut kefir or kombucha!

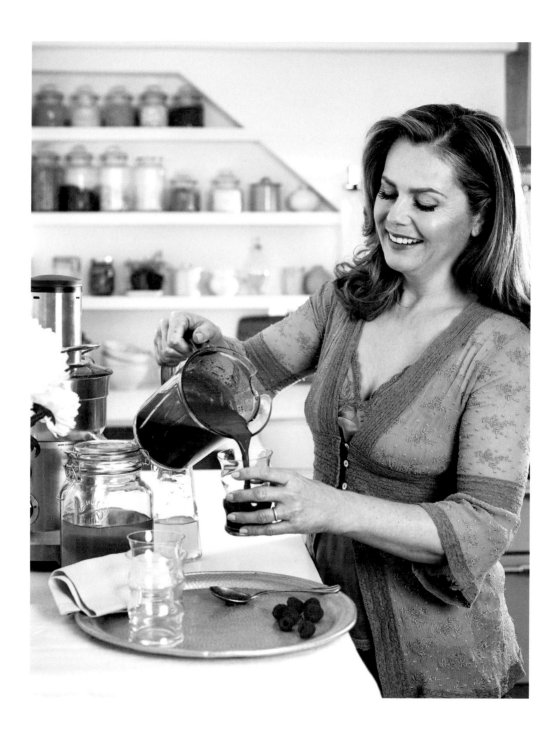

WEEK TWO:
Coming Clean

Week One kick-started the killing-off of an overgrowth of bad bugs and parasites that may have been lurking in your system. This week we'll be focusing on introducing healthy new habits to further cleanse and protect your microbiome, including a look at oral hygiene – important, since digestion begins in the mouth. How we brush our teeth and the types of products we use can affect the bacteria here, which in turn has a knock-on effect on what's going on lower down in our GI tract.

But first, let's look at our gut-health history and see how our upbringing and genetic make-up may have affected our microbiome. We can't change our past, but recognising and understanding how our gut health may have developed over our lifetime is one of the best bits of knowledge we can have with a view to better future health and wellbeing. It's also especially useful for those planning to have children, to start thinking about their future offspring's gut-health journey.

① Ages and stages

Birth and the first few weeks

The number of beneficial bacteria that can populate and proliferate in the gut of a newborn will largely determine whether or not that child develops allergies, intolerances, gut issues and even psychological disorders later on in life.

In the womb, babies have no gut bacteria of their own. They rely on the immune system of their mother to keep them healthy and strong, as the antibody IgG (immunoglobulin G) is transferred across the placenta to ward off infections.

It's only when babies travel down the birth canal that they become exposed to bacteria, which is a really important moment. Babies born by Caesarean don't get exposed to these microbes that live in the vagina, and therefore lose out. According to some findings, they can have weakened immune systems and also become more prone to asthma, allergies, food intolerances and even obesity later in life. C-section babies also tend to end up with more bacteria from the mother's skin, due to the way they come out and into their first human contact, with her torso. A greater understanding of the importance of vaginal delivery means it's becoming more common to take swabs from inside the mother's vagina during a C-section operation and wipe them over the baby's face at birth so they become inoculated with these protective bacteria.

AVOIDING ANTIBIOTICS: The early days of life are so crucial because they provide the opportunity to build strong foundations for the future. Antibiotics should be avoided unless absolutely necessary: a baby's immature GI tract has very few bacteria, so broad-spectrum antibiotics will kill off the majority of the newly colonising microbes, leaving the infant open to the possibility of more infection. Only use when essential.

WHY BREAST IS BEST: Giving an infant breast milk during the first days is also vital – some recommend 8–12 times a day or more. This is because early milk contains a substance called colostrum, which is packed with beneficial proteins and carbohydrates as well as antibodies to bolster the baby's immune system. This amazing, thick, sticky substance is only produced at the late stages of pregnancy and for the first few days, so it's vital to make the most of it. For example, a baby's gut is extremely permeable, but colostrum helps seal up the gaps, creating a protective barrier to stop foreign substances penetrating and causing allergic reactions to any unidentified particles in the mother's milk. It also has a laxative effect, so it helps newborns pass stools with ease.

The amount of colostrum in breast milk naturally decreases over the first fortnight after birth, when concentrations of these protective antibodies decrease, but the milk volume increases as the baby's stomach grows larger to accommodate more. However, even though the first weeks are the best in terms of immunity protection and strengthening, the disease-fighting properties remain throughout breastfeeding, so the longer it continues, the better.

Childhood

In 2015, a public health study showed that by the time they reach the age of eleven, a third of British children are overweight or obese. There's no doubt our processed diet has contributed to this, as was shown in a small study in 2010 comparing European children with some native to Africa. Scientists from the University of Florence compared the faecal matter of healthy European children with that of children from a rural village in Burkina Faso. The African children naturally ate a diet low in fat and animal protein and rich in starch and fibre from cereals, beans and other vegetables, similar to that of early humans. The European children, on the other hand, often ate a diet packed with sugar, animal fat and other calorie-dense foods – the kind of diet likely to lead to weight gain and other health problems.

To benefit the microbiome and help stave off obesity during childhood, the best foods to eat are lentils and grains, both of which are high in fibre and starches to feed the microbiome and prevent constipation, as well as all other types of vegetables and fruit – the whole fruit, not just the juice. Introducing these foods early to a child's diet helps them grow accustomed to a variety of tastes and textures – try to get as much variety into their diet as possible before the age of two, which is when most fussy eating habits tend to develop. Most children like yoghurts – they often prefer the fatty, creamy texture to that of crunchy foods – so feeding them plain live yoghurt is great for boosting good gut bacteria. If they don't like the taste, simply blitz it up with some low-sugar berries such as strawberries or blueberries.

The mix of microbes can vary a lot during early childhood and it's now that diversity is at its highest. Illness and all the new foods a child eats will cause shifts in the microbiome, so it's important to introduce as many foods as possible.

ANTIBIOTICS AND CHILDHOOD OBESITY: As I've stressed already, it's important too to keep antibiotic use to a minimum and, if possible, avoid giving them to children before the age of two, as this is when the gut microflora are still proliferating. However, around 70 per cent of children aged two and under are given antibiotics at least once. Those given them four times when under this age are far more likely to be obese by their fifth birthday. And repeated courses and large doses of antibiotics can have effects that may last years, or even a lifetime.

So many changes are taking place in the toddler brain and, interestingly, regressive-onset autism, when the child's development regresses, often occurs during this time, before the age of three. It's also the time when his or her microbiome is becoming fully established.

Teenagers

The gut microbiome continues to morph throughout our lives, and can become susceptible to disruption during the teenage years when hormones are flying around. It's a time when anxiety and depression, schizophrenia and eating disorders are most likely to occur. And in healthy adolescents too, without clinical psychiatric illness, it's likely there will be altered behaviour such as risk-taking, sensation-seeking, impulsivity and emotional instability. A diverse microbiome may keep your teen calmer, happier and less open to the effects of stress.

Avoiding foods full of additives, sugar and partially hydrogenated fats, such as most fast-food-chain meals, packaged meals in supermarkets and most biscuits, pastries and cakes, will help keep teens on an even keel when it comes to energy, focus and also feeling happier. It's worth noting that most teens are exposed to lots of fast-food advertising. The reward centre in the brains of adolescents shows a greater response to food advertising and fast-food logos compared to other types of adverts. What's more, teens are not as well equipped to forgo immediate treats in exchange for the promise of long-term good health. This is why it's important to talk to your children about eating a balanced diet and to set a good example yourself, because it not only helps them feel better and study more easily, it will also help them keep slim – usually a pretty good incentive!

The teenage years are also a time when pharmaceutical drugs may be offered to try to balance out hormone problems, such as the contraceptive pill to minimise heavy periods, or drugs to lessen the severity of acne. Short-term use of these medications can be very helpful here, but it's important to be aware of all the side effects, including those relating to gut health that are just becoming known. Eating well and learning to manage stress will both help keep teens' hormones healthy and balanced. And once acne is under control via prescription drugs, a focus on gut health can really help keep the skin clear.

MORE REASONS TO KISS

Young lovers can benefit from their new-found close contact for the good reason that swapping saliva during a romantic kiss exposes us to about 80 million individual bacteria! This could actually be a good thing, as scientists say it boosts our own immune system as we gain new strains of bacteria, thereby enabling us to fight off more infections – assuming our microbiome is in good shape in the first place.

Adulthood

During adulthood, although our microbiome is pretty stable, it still changes in response to illness, disease, antibiotics, fever, stress, injury, and also diet. But whatever happens, our population of microbes tends to shift back to our own regular baseline, largely set up in childhood.

HORMONES: For women, major events such as pregnancy and the menopause can cause even more shifts. Hormones also seem to affect our guts more than men's. Approximately a third of women experience GI symptoms during their period, and round 40 per cent with IBS say their menstrual cycle makes the IBS worse. This is probably due to fluctuations in ovarian hormones, which tend to cause bad cramps and GI symptoms.

STRESS: This can have detrimental effects on microbes. It may be brought on by anything from a stressful job or relationship, to juggling too many things, as tends to happen in midlife when there are not only children but also ageing parents to care for. The hormone cortisol is constantly elevated during times of chronic – that's to say, long-term – stress. Cortisol disrupts the balance of the gut bacteria, for example allowing colonies of candida yeast to overgrow. These feed off sugars, so are likely to have us reaching for cakes and sweet treats when we're feeling stressed, only making the problem worse. Recognising this can help us control it.

- **Take it easy:** Finding just 10 minutes a day to sit quietly, breathe slowly and calm your mind can significantly help to lower stress.
- **Eat well:** It's so important to eat well, in the same way that I advise for teenagers: lots of healthy fats, sulphur-rich cruciferous vegetables (broccoli, kale, cabbage) to support your liver, and alkalising your body with simple things such as having lemon juice in water first thing (yes, freshly squeezed lemon juice is alkalising), as well as eating a largely plant-based diet. Cutting out refined sugar is important too – studies now link excess sugar with the onset of Alzheimer's, as we're about to discover in the section on older age. Another way to stave off this brain disease is to stay a healthy weight. Research in America has shown that those who are overweight in their forties are at greater risk of developing Alzheimer's later on in life.

Older age

As we age, our immune systems can weaken, leading to more infections as well as an increased possibility of developing autoimmune diseases and cancer.

After sixty-five, the number of microbial species in our gut decreases, and those fewer species tend to show less diversity. Fortunately, prebiotics, probiotics and symbiotics (foods or supplements that contain both pre- and probiotics) have all been found to improve the immune response in older people.

A healthy gut may even be able to stave off degenerative diseases such as Alzheimer's. At the University of Perugia in Italy, scientists are looking at whether probiotics can alleviate memory loss. It's already known that the gut impacts the body in numerous ways other than the obvious, including cognitive functions such as learning, memory and decision-making, and many scientists now believe in a microbiota-driven gut–brain connection indicating activity between the central nervous system and the intestine.

Their theory is that probiotic supplements might help reduce the decline in age-related brain function, thanks to an experiment that found these good bacteria could impact our brain processes. And while life expectancy in general has improved in most developed countries, age-related diseases such as dementia are still a big concern. Scientists from the Institute of Agrochemistry and Food Technology in Spain say there is a significant relationship between gut microbes, diet and lifestyle among the elderly. Their research shows that probiotics and prebiotics given to older people can stimulate *Bifidobacterium* levels while decreasing the often harmful *Enterobacteriaceae*. Inflammation also lessened in the elderly individuals who were taking probiotics.

Even Parkinson's disease is now being linked to gut health. Reports out in summer 2015 reveal a possible link between the condition originating in the intestines and then slowly spreading up to the brain via the vagus nerve (see page 72). Further research has revealed a clear biological link between gut bacteria and Parkinson's disease.

Plenty of alternative healthcare practitioners advocate keeping your gut healthy in order to keep your brain sharp. In old age – in fact at any age – there are ways to help stave off brain-related diseases and improve overall health:

1. **Good fats:** Important throughout every stage of your life. Hormones are made from cholesterol, so healthy fats are vital, especially during the teenage years (and then again during the menopause). Omega-3s not only provide anti-inflammatory benefits but also help make sure hormones are being produced properly. One Omega-3 (DHA) is linked to slowing the progression of Alzheimer's disease. Avocados, oily fish, nuts and seeds are all good sources.

2. **Broccoli:** Broccoli, as well as other sulphur-rich vegetables such as cauliflower, turnips and kale, helps keep the liver healthy, which is important as this is the body's organ of detoxification.

3. **Ditch the sugar:** If you weren't already convinced to cut out the white stuff, sugar is now being linked to brain deterioration. In fact, Alzheimer's has been dubbed 'type 3 diabetes' by some because of the way high blood glucose levels and insulin resistance cause the brain to deteriorate. Healthier alternatives are the herb stevia, which has a very sweet taste, and Lakanto, whose main ingredient is monk fruit, popular in Japan as a low-sugar option.

4. **Flax seeds:** These help bring hormones into balance, thanks to their fibre and essential fatty acid content, and are great for good digestive health. They're packed with Omega-3s and also lignans, plant-based phytoestrogens that help regulate

oestrogen production, which is why they may be particularly good for growing girls and menopausal women. In the gut, lignans are converted by good bacteria into a form of oestrogen the body can use. Try sprinkling milled flax seeds onto cereal or salads.

5. **Butter:** Our brains need fat to function, and while butter was once vilified, now there are studies showing not only that it contributes to the healthy production of butyrate in our gut – a substance that's both anti-inflammatory and helps the gut produce new healthy cells – but that it can also help prevent Alzheimer's. Choose butter from cows grazed on forage and grass (look for the Free Range Dairy Pasture Promise label).

② Keep a food diary

Our bodies are unique and we react to foods in different ways. A food diary can help you keep track of any symptoms you may have. After each meal, in a diary, a notepad or an app on your phone, jot down all the foods you have eaten as well as how you feel. Include any symptoms you may have such as itchy skin, bloating, headaches – anything at all – and the times they occurred. Do this until the end of the six weeks, and you'll soon be able to see any patterns that emerge between the foods (and drinks) you ingest and how you feel.

Perhaps you'll notice that anything sugary always makes you bloated. Sadly, it's often the foods we eat the most and come to love that can cause us problems. This may be because they're feeding bad bacteria in our gut, and it's these that are causing our cravings – the sugar is satisfying the microbes, not us! And don't forget, they can influence our mind as well as our body.

Some may find they are sensitive to the FODMAP foods (Fermentable Oligosaccharides, Disaccharides, Monosaccharides and Polyols) – that is, ones that contain certain carbohydrates that cause bloating. So if you have IBS-type symptoms and can't seem to fathom the cause, it may be you have a tough time digesting some or all prebiotic foods, such as garlic, onions, leeks, artichokes, apples, beans, wheat and dairy products. Others may find that fruits and vegetables in the nightshade family – such as chillies, peppers, aubergines, strawberries and potatoes – cause irritation.

The important thing is to listen to your body. It's impossible to list foods that will definitely cause problems because we are all unique and it very much depends on the make-up of your gut bacteria. The best idea is to keep that food diary and track any symptoms. Then, if you suspect one food is causing the problem, cut it out for a full week and see whether that makes a difference. You can also get help with detecting the foods that are giving you trouble by visiting a dietitian, a nutritionist or a natural medicine practitioner who can assist you with an elimination diet, and/or find out which foods are the problem ones by carrying out blood tests or other kinds of food screening.

③ Oral hygiene

This whole microbiome thing isn't limited to our digestive system: as I suggested earlier, our mouth, too, houses a microbiome, which is intrinsically linked to the one in our gut. An estimated 700 different types of bacteria live in your mouth, most of which belong to the *Streptococcus* genus. Despite the negative association with a few of the strep bacteria (known for causing 'strep throat'), most are perfectly harmless and do a good job of fighting off invading bacteria.

Plaque, often thought of as the enemy, is actually a part of the mouth's microbiome, protecting our teeth and gums. It only gets thick, sticky and smelly, especially in the mornings, when we've eaten too many of the wrong foods and upset the gut's microbial balance. Rather than stripping it away as we've been taught to, we can instead restore a better microbial balance in our mouth so we don't produce as much plaque in the first place. Eating a more alkalising diet made up of plant-based foods rich in antioxidants can help here. Taking the food supplement CoQ10 is also thought to be beneficial. Most of us diligently brush twice a day with toothpastes that, according to some experts, are harming our oral microbiomes. 'Bacteria in the mouth keep you alive. If we were successful in eradicating all plaque … we would unleash ecological Armageddon because the bacteria in the mouth protect us from deadly viruses and bacteria in our environment,' says the New York 'rejuvenation dentist' Dr Gerry Curatola.

SOME TIPS FOR A HEALTHY ORAL MICROBIOME:

- **Check the ingredients**
  Chemicals found in most mouthwashes and toothpastes upset the balance of microbes inside your mouth. Avoid toothpastes and mouthwashes containing the gut-disrupting chemical triclosan and sodium lauryl sulfate (SLS), a known gum irritant. It's also best to avoid mouthwashes containing alcohol, as it's drying and kills beneficial bacteria.

- **Make your own mouthwash**
  Try making your own mouthwash with water and sage or peppermint. Simply steep a handful of fresh, clean sage or peppermint leaves (or a heaped teaspoon of the dried organic herb) in 200ml of freshly boiled filtered water (avoid tap water as this contains chlorine, which can also destroy friendly bacteria) and a teaspoon of salt. Keep in a clean screw-top jar and use within a week.

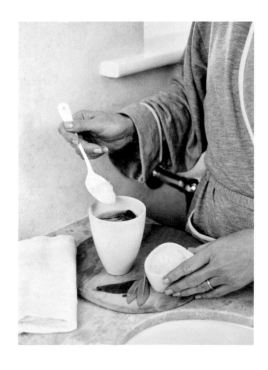

Rinse with a salt solution
You can also make a salt solution to use as a mouthwash. Just keep putting salt into filtered or spring water until the salt no longer dissolves at the bottom, meaning the water is now saturated. Use a few teaspoons of it in the morning to rinse your mouth after brushing.

Morning mouth rinse
Rinse your mouth with filtered or spring water as soon as you get up and before you have anything to drink. Keeping the mouth hydrated goes a long way to prevent bad breath from building up and is such a simple daily habit.

4 | Top up your stomach acid

The stomach is the most acidic environment in our body – an empty stomach should have a pH of around 1.5–3.5 (7.0 is neutral and anything above that is considered alkaline). The reason such high acidity is required is to properly digest food, especially proteins. This acidity is caused by the production of hydrochloric acid, also known as HCl, which helps us absorb vitamins and minerals.

A great health misunderstanding is that when we're suffering with heartburn we should reach for the antacids to lower our stomach acid. Despite depleting HCl, antacids can actually make matters worse over time. Because of this, many natural medicine practitioners are now prescribing HCl supplements. One such naturopath is Lucinda Miller, also known as the NatureDoc, who identifies around 30 per cent of the population over the age of sixty-five as having low stomach acid – a condition known as hypochlorhydria. 'Stress can also play a part in low HCl, as can deficiencies in zinc, calcium, magnesium, iron and vitamin B12,' she says. 'Deficiencies in these vitamins and minerals are often due to chronic stress, alcohol consumption and/or smoking, or just not eating enough foods rich in these nutrients.'

In cases of no stomach acid at all, a condition called achlorhydria, the pH is 6.5–7, which is the same as water and means the food that enters the stomach cannot be digested properly. This is sometimes found in seemingly healthy people who may have mental health conditions, severe mental fatigue, and even those who worry persistently – another reason for taking time out to relax.

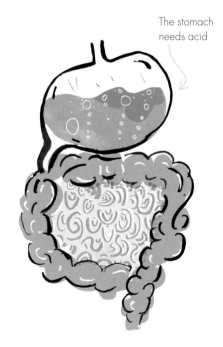

The stomach needs acid

Test yourself

Do you have low stomach acid?

You can work out whether you're probably lacking in HCl by looking at the following checklist devised by Lucinda Miller. Score 1 for each time you answer yes to the following symptoms:

- Bloating, belching, burning or wind immediately after and/or 45 minutes after eating
- Indigestion after eating
- Excess wind after eating
- Diarrhoea, constipation or both soon after eating
- Sense of fullness immediately after eating
- Nausea after taking supplements
- Persistent mucus in throat
- Iron deficiency
- Weak, flaking or cracked fingernails
- Dilated blood vessels in the cheeks and nose (rosacea)
- Spots, acne
- Undigested food in stools
- Itchy rectum
- Do you always eat in a rush?
- Do you chew your food properly?

If you scored 3 or more, it's likely you have low HCl and could benefit from taking a supplement or from naturally assisting your gut to produce more of it by following the suggestions overleaf.

How to top up

Encourage your stomach to produce more of its own stomach acid, naturally:

- Add lemon or lime juice to water and sip 30 minutes before your meal. Try not to consume any liquids while eating, though, as this further dilutes the stomach's acid.

- Add a tablespoon of raw apple cider vinegar or homemade Kombucha (see page 104) to a glass of warm water 30 minutes before each meal – drink through a straw to prevent damage to tooth enamel.

- Try taking Swedish bitters, a herbal elixir containing angelica root, aloe, myrrh, saffron, camphor and rhubarb root among other ingredients. It also contains essential oils. This elixir is said to soothe and disinfect the GI tract, improve kidney and liver function, boost bile production, restore your gut's natural pH balance and reduce bloating and gas. Take one teaspoonful diluted in a little water twice a day.

- Chew on bitter leaves such as rocket, chicory, endive, Little Gem lettuce, or drink lettuce, dandelion or gentian tea before each meal.

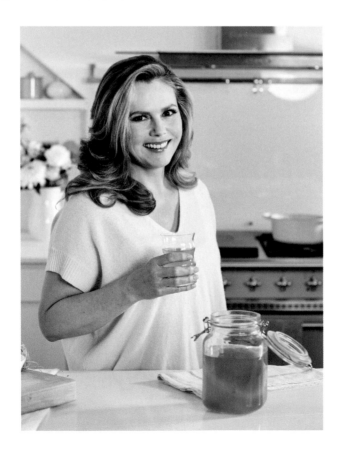

⑤ Soothe your skin

Just as we need to look after and bolster the beauty-boosting bacteria inside our gut, so we also need to protect the microbes that live on our skin. Our overzealous passion for clean, clear skin can lead to it being stripped of the microbes that actually keep our complexions smooth and blemish-free. I have long maintained that we shouldn't use anything that foams to clean our faces – and new research into how our skin's microbiome works backs this up.

For skin to stay strong and healthy, it needs to be mildly acidic – between pH 4.2 and 5.6. According to dermatological gut-health researcher Karen Sinclair Drake, 'When your skin is at the right pH, it allows certain microbes on it to communicate with your immune system. These messages go back and forth to give information about things such as your temperature, and whether you need to get ready to fight off an infection. It should naturally maintain this pH level thanks to lactic acid, which is produced when we sweat. In this optimum pH environment, beneficial bacteria can flourish that actually protect our skin.'

However, around 65 per cent of the population has alkaline skin, which is basically 'sick skin'. Sinclair Drake's study observing gut health and the skin reports that when skin is alkaline we lose good bacteria because they detach more easily, leaving the skin's surface drier, more brittle and more susceptible to sun damage and wrinkles.

CLEANSE FOR A HEALTHY COMPLEXION

The best way to keep skin healthily alkaline is to clean our faces not with soap or a foaming facial wash but with an oil-based cream cleanser. Using a creamy detergent-free cleanser or cleansing oil, simply removed with a warm, damp cotton muslin cloth or flannel, is by far the best way to maintain a clear, healthy complexion. Lactic acid is also a useful ingredient when it comes to skincare, and one of the easiest – yet most effective – ways to get the benefits from this is to apply live yoghurt directly to the skin. Simply rub a little plain, live – the key word here is live – yoghurt or milk kefir into clean skin two or three times a week. Gently massage across the face and neck for a few minutes using circular fingertip movements, then rinse away with warm water and pat the skin dry.

Plenty of us now take essential fatty acid supplements packed with Omega-3s and gamma-linolenic acid (GLA) to maintain a healthy skin, which can be very effective. However, the skin is usually the last organ to benefit from any essential nutrient, as the body circulates nutrients to all our vital organs before depositing any residues within our skin cells. This is why proper digestion and absorption are so essential to make the most of any skin-boosting supplements you take – otherwise, they may simply never reach the skin. If we don't absorb what we are eating well enough, whether it's food, drink or supplements, we won't reap the benefits – and the effects certainly won't show up on our skin. Good gut health gives skin a genuine healthy glow.

Make your own probiotic face mask

Half a ripe avocado
2 tbsp plain live yoghurt or milk kefir
1 tsp unprocessed (raw) runny honey

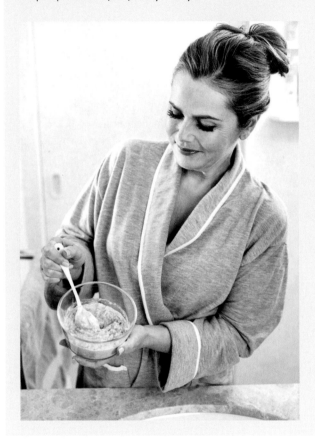

Simply mash the ingredients together to form a smooth paste and apply to freshly cleansed skin. Relax for 10–15 minutes (a soak in the bath is a useful time to do this) before rinsing away. The avocado remoisturises and provides natural vitamin E, the honey is purifying and moisturising, while the yoghurt or milk kefir contains lactoferrin to help boost beneficial bacteria and support healthy microbes on the skin. Those with breakouts or areas of inflammation can increase the effectiveness of this simple mask by stirring in the contents of a probiotic capsule.

GOOD-GUT CHECKLIST

1. **Stock up on anti-inflammatory foods**
   Dark leafy greens and herbs that promote detoxification such as those recommended in Week One help balance intestinal pH levels and ward off overgrowths of bad bacteria.

2. **Do away with antibacterial oral products**
   Synthetic toothpastes and mouthwashes can actually strip away the naturally helpful bacteria in your mouth. Try using brands with no SLS, antibacterial ingredients or alcohol. Switch to more naturally based brands and try making your own herb or salt mouth rinse.

3. **Increase your stomach acid**
   An easy way to encourage better digestion is to take a teaspoonful of raw apple cider vinegar in water before each meal. The acid kick-starts your digestive juices. If you struggle with heavy proteins, consider taking an HCl supplement with each meat-based meal – at least until your body is producing enough of its own.

4. **Love your lactoferrin**
   Skin prone to acne and spotty breakouts may well benefit from this protein present in the lactic acid of fermented dairy produce, such as live yoghurt, buttermilk and sour cream. It has clinically proven antimicrobial and anti-inflammatory properties, especially when combined with a low GI/GL (glycaemic index or glycaemic load) diet.

5. **Keep up the kefir**
   Studies show kefir, made from fermented milk, to be one of the most valuable gut-health builders. Homemade versions generally contain many more strains of beneficial bacteria than shop-bought, see page 106. Useful for both internal and external use (add to face masks).

WEEK THREE:
Healing and Repopulation

This week we'll look at some of the many different strains of bacteria and how they can benefit a diverse range of conditions, as well as considering which probiotic foods to prioritise to help your gut on its way to becoming so much healthier and happier. Bacterial strains can change in as little as a few weeks with the right foods, drinks and lifestyle choices, so there's lots we can all do, starting today, to boost these bacteria to better health.

Beneficial bacteria can come from many different sources, from straightforward supplements of probiotics to foods and drinks rich in gut-boosting bacteria. Eating fermented and cultured food also boosts our supplies, and we can even obtain gut-friendly organisms from traces of soil dirt.

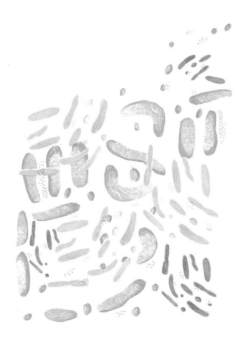

① Brush up on your bacteria

Back in the late nineteenth century, microbiologists first identified microflora in the guts of healthy people that differed from those found in people who were sick. They named these beneficial microflora 'probiotics' – 'pro' meaning 'for', and 'biotics' from the Greek word meaning 'life' – as they were proven to make us healthier. Numerous studies over the past few decades, and especially in the last five years, have confirmed the important role probiotics play as part of a healthy diet. In short, they create a natural barrier against infection and keep our whole body strong, especially our immune system.

Some of the most studied benefits of probiotics include:

- Strengthening the immune system so we're better able to fight off infection.

- Controlling or alleviating inflammatory bowel disease (IBD) as well as irritable bowel syndrome (IBS).

- Lessening food allergies in children.

- Lowering blood cholesterol levels.

- Reducing the incidence of antibiotic-related and traveller's diarrhoea.

- Helping us better digest milk products (in the case of the *Lactobacillus* strains).

- Improving the pH, i.e. increasing the level of acidity, of our intestines so that bad bacteria and viruses are killed off.

LEARNING THE LINGO

The first word of a bacterium's name is the genus, which is the group to which the bacteria belong, e.g. *Streptococcus*. The second word refers to the species, which is the individual type of bacterium, e.g. *Lactobacillus rhamnosus*. If letters or numbers follow, this refers to the strain, of which there are often many, or it can be a differentiation of the species. For example: *Lactobacillus acidophilus* NCFM – *Lactobacillus* is the genus, *acidophilus* is the species, and NCFM is the particular strain. The two most common types of probiotic are the *Lactobacillus* and *Bifidobacterium* groups (or genera, the plural of genus).

② A bug's life

Probiotic supplements are hugely helpful in repopulating our microbiome, so let's put these microbes under the microscope. While there is research going on into individual strains and what they can do, for now most natural health practitioners recommend taking a supplement containing as many types of bacteria as possible, as diversity is the key to good health. The more good-gut bugs we have, the fewer bad ones can get a look-in. I look for supplements that contain at least ten strains – and try to include all of those listed below for at least some of the time. In the future, we can expect to see better identification and/or genetically engineered probiotics targeting specific diseases.

Lactobacillus acidophilus: Found commonly and abundantly in live yoghurt, this bacterium is often added to dietary supplements as it survives transit through the gut. It's been linked with improved intestinal health, stronger immunity, better absorption of nutrients, a reduction in lactose intolerance, less severe allergies, and even a reduced risk of colon cancer (albeit in an animal study).

Lactobacillus bulgaricus: This hardy strain has been shown to survive the acidic environment of the stomach. It's most commonly found in Bulgarian yoghurt and Swiss cheese and has the ability to reduce infections by altering the pH of our gut to kill pathogens and produce its own immune-boosting natural antibiotics. It may be a reason why those who eat Swiss dairy products from mountain-flower-grazed dairy cows are better protected against disease (the so-called Swiss Alpine Paradox).

Lactobacillus plantarum: This type is known to reduce bloating, flatulence and pain in those with IBS, and has also been shown to help boost the immune system in infants. On that note, it might be useful for your little ones, as one study showed it reduced the number of bouts of diarrhoea at daycare centres when given to only half of the children. It's also been found to reduce inflammation of the bowel, as well as reducing minor intestinal bacterial overgrowth (SIBO) in children.

Lactobacillus reuteri: This type of bacteria is proven to shorten the duration of acute gastroenteritis with diarrhoea. And when it comes to vaginal thrush, a particular strain of *L. reuteri*, RC-14, together with *L. rhamnosus* GR-1, has been shown to help reduce the overgrowth of candida. Both bacteria are also shown to help minimise bacterial vaginosis (BV) when combined with traditional antibiotic treatment (metronidazole).

Lactobacillus rhamnosus: A key bacterium for good gut health as well as whole-body wellness, *L. rhamnosus* survives stomach acid and can protect the stomach lining. In one trial, yoghurt containing the strain *L. rhamnosus* GG cleared up a type of bad bacteria shown to be resistant to the antibiotic vancomycin, which is often prescribed for acute diarrhoea. Like *Lactobacillus reuteri* above, it's also been used to reduce thrush and BV and can boost immunity against certain infections. It's also beneficial for our mental health, able to reduce anxiety by bringing down stress hormones and regulating GABA, a mood-boosting neurotransmitter. In terms of childhood benefits, fermented milk containing *L. rhamnosus* GG has been found to shorten the duration of diarrhoea in children with an upset stomach due to rotavirus.

Bifidobacterium animalis lactis: *B. lactis* is a hardy probiotic shown to stay active for a long time and improve gut health by competing with bad bacteria for food sources – and winning! This makes it instrumental in reducing pathogens, especially in cases where antibiotics have caused harmful strains to multiply.

Bifidobacterium bifidum: This is the most dominant probiotic found in the guts of infants and in the large intestines of most adults. It supports the production of vitamins, inhibits bad bacteria, supports the immune system and also helps prevent diarrhoea. In a study on healthy full-term babies, when *B. bifidum* was added to formula milk it provided similar health benefits to breast milk.

Bifidobacterium breve: This is one of the most predominant bacteria found inside the guts of newborn babies, and comes from the mother's milk. *B. breve* helps babies digest oligosaccharides (a type of carbohydrate) found in breast milk. It's less abundant in adults and declines as we age, possibly due to antibiotic use as it's been found to be easily killed off by the drugs. *B. breve* is most important for the digestion of many foods, including tough plant fibres and a number of complex carbohydrates, as well as maintaining the health of the intestines and warding off *E. coli* and other pathogens. Make sure your probiotic supplement includes it.

Streptococcus thermophilus: This is a lactic acid bacterium and is often found in fermented milk, cheese and yoghurt, helping break down the lactose (milk sugar). In fact, *S. thermophilus* is regularly used as a dairy starter, meaning it kick-starts the fermentation process. However, pasturisation destroys this type of probiotic, so using raw milk as your dairy starter and eating unpasteurised cheese are the best food sources. *S. thermophilus* has also been found to help prevent bad bacteria from attaching to the lining of our gut, to stimulate disease-fighting cells and reduce the amount of nitrites in the body, which in some cases have been linked to cancer. One strain, *S. thermophilus* TH-4, is currently undergoing research as to its potential in preventing severe inflammation of the small intestine, which can happen during chemotherapy.

Akkermansia muciniphila: Not often included in multi-strain probiotics, *A. muciniphila* could be the future when it comes to maintaining a healthy weight. It's been found that the more of this bacterium you have, the leaner you're likely to be. Around 4 per cent of a slim person's microbiome comes from this species; whereas those who are overweight or obese hardly have any. The reason it helps keep weight off is because it lives on the thick layer of mucus that coats the lining of your gut, forming a barrier. The less *A. muciniphila* you have, the thinner this mucus layer may be; therefore, the more likely it is that bacteria, good or bad, will make it through to your bloodstream. A 2013 study of mice found that supplementing with *A. muciniphila* could reduce the blood levels of unhealthy lipopolysaccharides (LPS) and therefore lead to weight loss.

③ Be a savvy probiotic shopper

There are now hundreds of probiotic supplements available to buy both in health food shops and online. Which ones should we choose? Well, the number of different strains a probiotic supplement contains is important. As I mentioned, you want diversity – look for a multi-strain with a minimum of ten different types, and the number of microbes counted in the billions, not millions. Also, choose a product that says it is guaranteed to survive high stomach acid. You might also be interested to know that most probiotics are of animal origin; that is, the bacteria started life in the stomach of an animal (or even a human) and were then cultured in a test tube to create millions and billions of them.

Liquids or powders?

The two main types of delivery method are freeze-dried probiotics put into capsules (the most common type) or sachets, and liquids containing live strains. Critics of freeze-drying say not all the bacteria are alive when they reach the gut, so we may be getting far fewer of them than is stated on the packet – which is why it's so important to look for a high-strength product to begin with. And if the bacteria are alive, they might not make it through our acidic stomach to the large intestine, which they do need to reach in order to do any good. Others swear by freeze-dried capsules and powders (myself included) as they see real results from taking them. Some doctors don't believe in supplements at all, suggesting it's far better to eat foods rich in probiotics and prebiotics to naturally boost our own levels of good-gut bacteria. Others, such as Dr Raphael Kellman, founder of the Microbiome Medicine Summit, advocate taking supplements as an 'insurance policy', which seems a sensible and balanced approach.

If you do take a daily probiotic (as I do), take it first thing on an empty stomach and swallow with water. This minimises the amount of stomach acid present that could reduce its effectiveness. Last thing at night is also a good option, if your stomach is empty.

STORAGE

When it comes to storage, always follow the advice on the packet, as some probiotics need to be refrigerated, while the makers of some freeze-dried versions claim their products don't. To be safe, I always keep mine cool or in the fridge.

SOIL-BASED PROBIOTICS

We all know spending time in natural surroundings is good for our mind, body and soul. Exercising in the great outdoors helps keep us fit and well, and now scientists are discovering another great reason to interact, perhaps more intimately, with nature.

The earth is teeming with tiny organisms that live in the soil, which help plants grow strong and healthy – without them they'd die of malnutrition or perish from viruses. Often referred to as soil-based organisms (SBOs) or soil-based probiotics, these bacteria could support our health in a number of ways. SBOs seem to improve conditions in our large intestine, helping to create B vitamins – which we need for energy, among other things – and other important antioxidants. However, SBOs are spores that come from the ground and more research is needed as to whether taking supplements could be beneficial. For now, stick to tiny traces of soil on local fruit and veg, as these will be less alien to your own personal microbiome.

4 Soil health

Speaking of soil-based organisms, there's a growing collective of farmers, growers, health practitioners and researchers advocating that we should really get back to nature – quite literally – where gut health is concerned, by interacting with microbes found naturally in and on the earth. It's something of a backlash against the super-sterile environments most of us have grown up in and become accustomed to, with our antibacterial sprays, soaps and wipes always at the ready to disinfect every surface of our homes as well as ourselves. 'Increasing your exposure to microbes from dirt can be a good way to bring more diversity to your gut bacteria,' says Dr Josh Axe, the natural nutrition practitioner I mentioned earlier (page 30).

This brings me to homegrown fruit and veg. From having an allotment to owning even just a tiny space of soil, growing your own veg can not only save you money, it may also help improve your health. Fruit and veg plucked straight from a bush or tree or out of the ground, grown without pesticides or artificial fertilisers, offer us numerous health benefits. We ingest all the protective microbes living on the surface of the fruit or veg's skin. These microbes are what keep produce healthy and fresh as it grows. So, when you eat a fruit directly from the plant you'll also be tucking into millions of microbes that are good for you too. If you can't grow your own, shopping at a local farmers' market is the next-best thing, or selecting your own unwashed produce from the organic section of the supermarket.

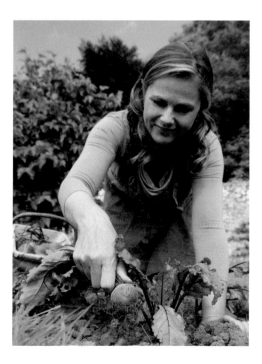

Try this:

- **Make a herb garden:** One of the easiest ways to grow your own produce, no matter how much space you have, is to plant up a pot with herbs. If you don't want to propagate your own (which takes some time), you can easily buy ready-grown herbs from the supermarket. Windowsill herbs grow all year round to supply fresh leaves week on week.

- **Keep a bit of dirt:** If your fruit and veg are organic, then don't worry about removing every single speck of earth – it could be full of health-giving organisms! It won't have been subjected to pesticides or to post-harvest herbicide sprays, which means you can loosely cold-wash your fruit and veg and still maintain some of the beneficial microbes. What's more, most of the friendly fibres that feed good-gut bugs are found directly under the skins of fruits, so don't peel. However, use caution if they've been picked from a plant growing on or near ground that cats, dogs or foxes frequent, as their faeces may be in the soil, which can give rise to toxoplasmosis and other dangerous infections.

- **Get out into the garden:** Connecting to the earth, touching it with your bare hands, is proven to be good for your health as you're connecting with millions of bacteria – so go out there and pot on some plants, dig up weeds or mow the lawn.

- **Take off your shoes:** We de-stress our whole body when we walk barefoot on the grass, soil or sand.

⑤ Love your bugs

One of the best ways to encourage the growth of all the good bacteria already inside us is to eat a diet rich in what are called 'prebiotics'. The difference between 'pro' and 'pre' is that probiotics are bacteria and yeasts, whereas prebiotics are (generally) foods that act as foods for the probiotics, especially *Lactobacillus* and *Bifidobacterium*, and help them multiply. Most prebiotics are found in vegetables, fruits, pulses and milks and are made up of indigestible fibres that can only be eaten up by the microbes in our gut.

All these indigestible fibres are good for gut health. For example, inulin, which is most often sourced from the root of the chicory plant, is able to boost digestion, alleviate constipation thanks to its ability to absorb lots of water, curb our appetite, lower bad (LDL) cholesterol, keep our blood sugar low and also help us absorb calcium. A wonder-plant indeed (and you'll find several delicious ways to cook it in Part Two).

Some of the main vegetable sources of prebiotics are:

- Garlic, onions, leeks and chives
- Asparagus
- Globe artichoke
- Green apples
- Fennel bulb
- Dandelion root
- Chicory root
- Peas
- Avocado

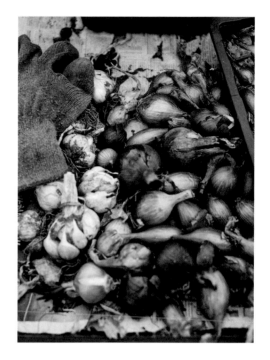

NOTE: The above are all FODMAP foods, which can trigger excess gas and bloating in those with dysbiosis, and many are included in the recipes in Part Two. But I've listed below some key ingredients that you may want to include a little of in your meals so as to get an extra boost of prebiotics.

Apple cider vinegar

Apple cider vinegar is a bit of a cure-all for the gut. Not only is it a prebiotic that helps feed our good bacteria, it's also rich in potassium, a mineral most of us are often low in if we eat too much salt (sodium competes with potassium in the body).

Encourage good digestion
Add a splash of the vinegar to water and drink it just before meals.

Always go raw
If you don't make your own (see page 102), check the label says 'unpasteurised' or 'raw' as this means it still contains 'the mother', which is another way of saying parts of the original ferment that contains pectin, trace minerals, beneficial bacteria and enzymes,

all of which will be floating in a sediment at the bottom. Seeing sediment is good!

Stop the snack attack
Next time you're tempted to wolf down an entire packet of biscuits, drink a small glass of water containing a teaspoon of apple cider vinegar – it really can help to lessen your sugar cravings.

Raw honey

Honey from a beekeeper near where you live almost certainly won't have been pasteurised (heat-treated), meaning it's still 'raw'. Increasingly, shops too are selling raw honey, so it's worth looking out for. The raw variety can contain more than 200 natural forms of pollen and microbes, almost all of which are good for our gut health. (Some raw honey may contain botulism spores that are very dangerous for babies, which is why honey must not be given to those under one year of age because they have not developed enough stomach acid to neutralise it.) Genuine raw honey contains the living form of the immune-boosting probiotic *Lactobacillus kunkeei*. The best way to identify raw honey is to buy a jar from a local beekeeper, or check that the label says 'unprocessed' and mentions the location of the beehives, for provenance.

- Try a teaspoon of raw honey on porridge or add it to largely veg-based smoothies, for sweetness.

- I treat myself to a teaspoonful of raw honey as a sweet-treat pick-me-up instead of reaching for junk confectionery.

Medicinal mushrooms

Forget whatever Dougal was taking on *The Magic Roundabout*, here I'm talking about fungi such as shiitake, cordyceps, turkey tail, reishi and lion's mane – all rather exotic-sounding mushrooms. These too have prebiotic qualities and are popular in Chinese and Japanese cooking, where they're added to miso bone broths, another fantastic gut healer.

CORDYCEPS: Only found in mountainous regions at altitudes of more than 3,800 metres above sea level. A different species from most fungi, they have incredible healing powers and when dried out they can be ground up into an extremely potent powder. Benefits include reducing coughs and colds as well as inflammation and tissue damage, alleviating stress or fatigue, and increasing energy levels and immunity.

SHIITAKE: These fungi are a great addition to any soup, stew or broth, thanks to their meaty texture. Healthwise they're rich in B vitamins and can help fight cancer cells, cardiovascular disease and infections thanks to their antiviral, antibacterial and antifungal properties. They contain all eight amino acids (proteins), which is why they're so good for those avoiding meat, and they are even reputed to have a fat-reducing effect.

REISHI: These mushrooms help to increase the levels of T-cells (a kind of lymphocyte) in our immune system, thanks to their large amounts of beta-glucans, sugars found in the cell walls of not only fungi but also bacteria, yeasts, algae, lichen, oats and barley. This boost to the T-cell count helps relieve symptoms related to autoimmune disorders. Given their other proven benefits – alleviating arthritis and muscle ache as well as improving focus and memory, plus de-stressing and aiding sleep – these little mushrooms really are all-round health marvels.

- **Add to stews:** It's easy to add a handful of the raw or dried mushrooms to a stew or broth to bring immunity-boosting benefits.

- **Try an extract:** Dried mushrooms including reishi, oyster, cep and shiitake are all available in the form of powders. Use them in cooking or add to hot water to make a tea. However, when looking for a powder, make sure it states that it's an 'extract'. These are heated to high temperatures along with an alcohol solution. The process breaks down the chitin content in the mushrooms, thereby unlocking their beneficial medicinal substances. Mushroom powders that are simply ground up and haven't been extracted won't be as bioavailable, i.e. your body won't absorb the beneficial medicinal nutrients so well. Extracts naturally tend to be more expensive, as extracting is a more labour-intensive process, but it means you'll be guaranteed to receive more of the benefits. However, even powders that are not extracts, as well as regular whole mushrooms, are still good for our digestion because chitin is a beneficial gut-friendly dietary fibre.

GOOD-GUT CHECKLIST

1. **Take a daily probiotic**
   Although it won't undo an unhealthy diet, taking a multi-strain probiotic each day is a useful insurance policy alongside a diet filled with fresh and fermented foods. It can also help speed up the transit time of food and waste matter passing through your body, easing and regulating bowel movements.

2. **Drink fermented beverages**
   Why not wash down your probiotics with a zingy kombucha shot or a glass of milk kefir? Also, use water kefir as the basis for probiotic-packed milkshakes and smoothies. Concentrated lacto fermented whey is also rich in *Lactobacillus* and can be added to water, juice and smoothies.

3. **Go organic**
   Buy fresh produce from farmers' markets or look in supermarkets for loose organic fruit and veg that have yet to be scrubbed clean. Again, you'll get those healthy soil-based bacteria that help improve digestive and immune functions. With your veg, loosely rinse them under the tap to remove the visible soil. A few tiny particles will be left behind in the crevices – but this is OK!

4. **Antibiotic antidote**
   Don't forget to take a probiotic supplement alongside any antibiotics. The two strains shown to be the most beneficial here are *L. acidophilus* and *L. rhamnosus*.

NOTE: Some fermented foods and drinks can be a trigger for those with migraine.

WEEK FOUR:
Nourish

By now, the chances are you'll be feeling lighter, brighter and far more energised! But do go easy on yourself if you're not – clearing away the bad bugs to make way for the new can make us feel temporarily worse. Whether you're feeling great or a bit under the weather, this week we'll focus on a few more interesting new ways we can nourish and soothe our digestion with probiotic supplements and foods to help restore and heal.

You can expect to see some significant changes to the way you look and feel during this week. It's also the perfect time to start making some of my best and most nourishing bone broth recipes (see pages 66–67).

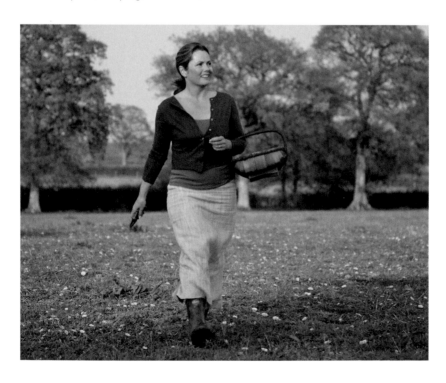

① Magnesium

The mighty mineral magnesium is good for helping us to relax, but it also goes far further than this: it plays a vital role in many bodily functions, including regulating blood sugar, keeping our heart beating healthily, forming bones and teeth, and promoting healthy bowel function.

- Dark leafy greens, brown rice, beans, wholegrains, nuts and even dark chocolate (minimum 70 per cent cocoa solids) are some of the best food sources of magnesium, so have at least some of these each day.

- Other foods rich in magnesium include seaweed, basil and coriander, pumpkin seeds and linseed (flax seed), unsweetened cocoa powder and almond butter. These are all excellent additions to smoothies, except perhaps the seaweed, which you could chop up and add to stir-fries or sprinkle on veggies instead.

- If you suspect you might be low in magnesium – frequent cramps, spasms or abnormal heart rhythms are symptoms – opt for a powdered magnesium citrate stirred into water or added to a herbal tea. Look for versions blended with calcium, as we need a balance of both minerals for proper muscle contraction and relaxation, including a healthy heartbeat.

If you do take a supplement, consider adding vitamins K2 and D alongside, as these work synergistically with magnesium. Overdosing on one can lead to a deficiency in another, so check with a nutritionist if you're unsure of the best amounts for you.

A MAGNESIUM BATH

As well as topping up on magnesium in our diet, there's another very nice way to maximise our magnesium intake which also helps to de-stress, and that's to have a relaxing bath with a few large handfuls of magnesium chloride salts. More effective and absorbable than Epsom salts (which are made of magnesium sulphate), magnesium chloride can bring real relief at the end of a busy day. Follow the directions on the packet and soak for at least 10–15 minutes before getting out of the bath and patting your skin dry.

② Good-gut supplements

Once our gut is cleansed and repopulated with beneficial bacteria, we can look to support it with some additional help.

Glutathione – the master detoxifier

Produced naturally by our liver, glutathione is a powerful antioxidant consisting of three key amino acids, and it's deemed by many to be the 'master detoxifier'. It gets this reputation because it can help prevent cell damage, build and repair tissues and contribute to maintaining a strong immune system. But it's not only a human substance – fruits, vegetables and animals make it too. Glutathione is used by the medical profession to alleviate all kinds of conditions, from cataracts and asthma to slowing ageing, preventing heart disease, staving off chronic fatigue syndrome and helping cancer patients regain their strength. The list is almost endless. But you needn't wait to get critically ill to take it. Everyone could probably benefit from a good dose of glutathione and we can encourage our body to produce more of its own, naturally, by eating a well-balanced diet, with a focus on the following foods:

- **Cruciferous vegetables** such as broccoli, kale, Brussels sprouts, cabbage, cauliflower and radishes.

- **Folate-rich foods** such as liver (one of the best sources), lentils, pinto beans, asparagus and black-eyed beans.

- **Selenium-rich foods** including brazil nuts, which are the best source: just 6–8 nuts provide all your daily selenium needs. Other sources include yellow-fin tuna, halibut, sardines and grass-fed beef.

- **Vitamin C-rich foods** such as kiwi fruits, berries, oranges and kale.

- **Vitamin E-rich foods** including almonds, spinach, avocado, sunflower seeds – and perhaps consider an evening primrose oil supplement too (choose one containing the Rigel seed variety).

MARVELLOUS MICRO-ALGAE

As well as being protein-packed, both chlorella and spirulina are fabulous all-round detoxifiers. Seen under the microscope, chlorella is flat and smooth, providing more surface area for mopping up toxins, bad bugs and heavy metals as it goes around the body, a bit like a magnet, moving them on through our colon or bladder to be safely excreted. Spirulina is a complete protein source, with all eight essential amino acids in their proper ratios, so is excellent for vegans and vegetarians alike. Add a teaspoon of these dark-green wonder powders to juice or to a smoothie – you'll definitely want to sweeten them, though, as they smell (and taste) a little too much like pond water! When buying chlorella, choose a variety described on the label as 'cracked [broken] cell wall', for greater absorption properties.

Liquorice root

Also known by its Latin name of *Glycyrrhiza glabra*, liquorice is a healing spice that has been used for centuries to soothe various digestive complaints, including ulcers, heartburn, colic and chronic gastritis (inflammation of the stomach lining). The flavonoid-rich extract is both antioxidant and anti-inflammatory, and can help kill off the pathogenic bacterium *Helicobacter pylori*, making it an excellent good-gut spice. It also adds an aromatically sweet taste to teas, and you'll often find commercial blends containing both cinnamon and liquorice.

Aloe vera

The gel from deep inside the leaves of this succulent plant has antibacterial, antifungal and antiviral properties. You may have used it on your skin after getting a little too much sun, and those same soothing properties can be felt inside your body too as the gel, a powerful anti-inflammatory, gets to work. Squeeze it directly from the plant's fat, juicy leaves – choose stems that are thick and at least 18 inches long. Or you can buy bottled sap and juice from health food stores. There are many brands out there, so check the labels to make sure you're getting a completely pure product, not one diluted with additives.

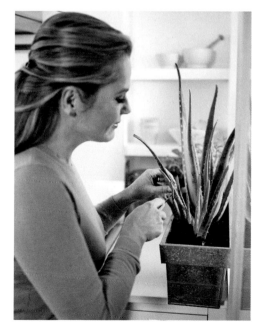

Slippery elm

This species of elm native to North America has been used for centuries in tummy tinctures. It's not the leaves but the inner bark that's dried and powdered for use in medicines. Slippery elm is traditionally taken to calm stomach upsets, including diarrhoea, as it produces a slippery mucilage when added to water, which helps to line and protect the gut wall.

Slippery elm also stimulates the nerve endings in the GI tract, prompting a mucus secretion that's also protective. Although a firm favourite with herbalists, there are scant scientific studies on this remedy, despite plenty of anecdotal evidence. If you buy it as a tincture, take around 5ml three times a day, or make your own tea by pouring two cups of boiling water over two teaspoons of powdered bark, then leave it to steep for up to five minutes. It's recommended that you drink a cupful three times a day, two hours before or after other herbs or medications you may be taking.

A SAFETY NOTE: **Pregnant women and those with a weakened immune system should avoid slippery elm.**

 # Say yes to exercise!

The reasons for taking regular exercise are plentiful, and you'll be pleased to know improved gut health is yet another benefit to add to the list. Why? Any type of movement, especially anything that involves jumping, running or dancing, helps encourage the smooth passage of food and waste through our intestines. After all, we can take all the healing herbs in the world and eat a super-healthy diet, but if we don't also combine that with movement, our body will have a hard time making its own 'movements', if you see what I mean.

Sweating as a result of exercise also means you're likely to increase your water intake, and that can improve bowel function too. But whether you're having problems going to the loo or not, exercising and upping your water intake will improve the frequency of your bowel movements and make them easier. Feeling stressed can also exacerbate constipation. Exercise not only gets things moving, it helps improve our mental wellbeing too, so it's a win-win all round.

HIGH-INTENSITY INTERVAL TRAINING: Bursts of high-intensity interval training (HIIT) constitute one of the latest fitness regimes. This is where you exercise flat out for 30 seconds, whether on a bike, doing star jumps or just jogging like mad on the spot. It's not only excellent for our cardio health and proven to burn more fat than steady-state exercise such as a half-hour jog, it also encourages proper elimination later as the movement shakes things up and encourages peristalsis (motility of the intestines). And the great thing about HIIT is that it need only take 5–10 minutes each day, meaning you can stay fit even if you're pushed for time.

WALKING: If fast and furious isn't your style, then you'll be pleased to know a walk in the park can be equally effective. The steady, rhythmic movement of taking step after step – especially if you up the speed to the point where you're slightly out of breath – will also encourage better digestion. My personal favourite is Nordic walking, using poles to stride out and build better upper-body strength as well as increase aerobic activity by boosting the heart rate.

YOGA: Of course, it's an amazing set of stretches for our body, and that includes our gut. The sheer variety of twisting poses, inversions and asanas that encourage us to reach for the sky and beyond gives our midriff and intestines an excellent internal workout.

PILATES: With similar benefits to yoga but with more focus on our inner core. Our muscles become toned and, in the process, stimulate our digestive organs. One of the basics of Pilates is to strengthen the transversus abdominis – a thin sheet of muscles that sits deep within our body and wraps around our pelvic organs like a corset. This muscle contracts in almost all Pilates moves, especially all the ones where you start from a lying-down, face-up position (supine) and pull your body up off the floor. The often dreaded 'hundred' move (level 2) involves raising the head, neck, shoulders and legs off the ground and pulsing the arms 100 times before lowering your body back down and is highly effective for promoting core strength as well as a boost for good gut health.

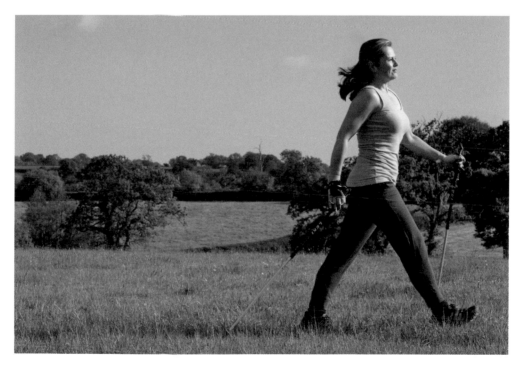

Nordic walking helps get the gut moving

Soothe with bone broth

You're probably used to thinking about collagen in relation to skincare as it's been a popular skincare ingredient for many years (except for vegetarian product ranges, being animal-derived). But did you know it's just as essential for our gut health? One of the best ways to help heal and seal our gut lining is with bone broth as, derived from animal bones or fish skins, it's naturally rich in collagen.

This easy-to-digest liquid can be either used as a stock for other recipes such as stews, or made into a simple soup by lightly boiling some veggies in with it. Try having it for your evening meal so your body doesn't have to work too hard to digest overnight – it should improve your quality of sleep too. I often make my batch by boiling up bones on a Sunday night, especially after serving a roast for lunch, then I keep some in the fridge for the week and freeze any left over.

If you're a vegetarian searching for amino acids you can try asparagus and beetroot, but the best source, in my opinion, is sea veg – especially spirulina as it contains gut-healing glutamine. You can also make veggie broths containing shiitake mushrooms, organic miso and fermented soy products.

Make your own beef bone broth

MAKES ABOUT 2 LITRES
PREP: ABOUT 6 HOURS

2kg organic grass-fed beef bones (buy cheaply from butcher or farm shop)
Sea salt and freshly ground black pepper

4 carrots, peeled and roughly chopped
1 onion, roughly chopped
1 bay leaf

Preheat the oven to 200°C/400°F/Gas Mark 6. Put the beef bones into a roasting tin, season with the sea salt and freshly ground black pepper, then tuck in half the carrots and half the onion and put in the oven for about 40 minutes or until the bones start to turn golden.

Remove from the oven and put the bones in a large stockpot along with the bay leaf and the remaining carrots and onion. Fill up with water to cover and bring to the boil, then simmer with the lid on for about 4–5 hours, skimming away any scum from the top of the pot. Remove from the heat and leave to cool completely.

When cold, spoon away the fat and strain the broth into a sealed container, and keep in the fridge for up to 2 weeks.

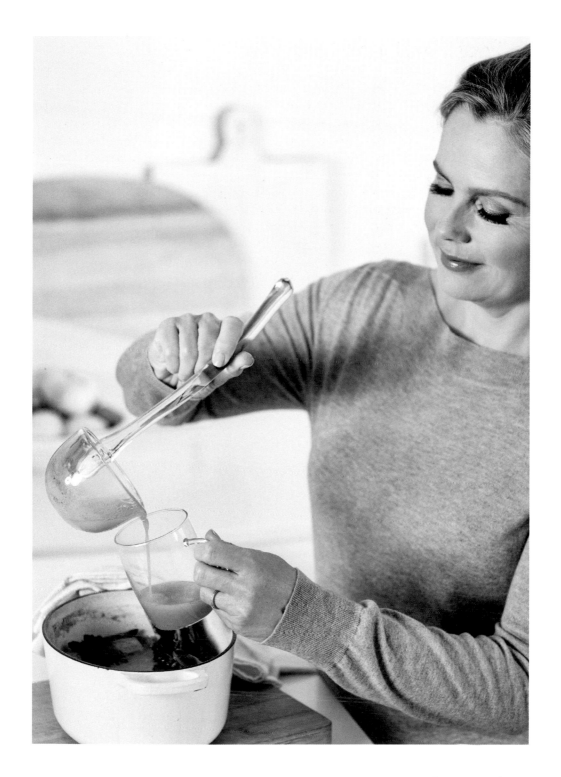

⑤ Reduce stress and sleep well

Sleep is crucial for both our brains and our bodies to rest and regenerate. And now it's known that our microbiome may affect not only how well we sleep but also our weight. For example, one study showed how jet lag caused a disruption to the microbiome which affected the circadian rhythm – the sleep–wake cycle. The microbes were thrown out of kilter by the new time zone and eating pattern, which led to dysbiosis – an unbalanced microbiome, described earlier – and glucose intolerance, which in turn resulted in weight gain.

Shift workers can experience these problems and find it difficult to manage their weight. It's therefore important to go to bed around the same time each evening when possible, as this will support good gut health.

- **Say no to blue light**
  Start to unwind at around 9 p.m. each night and switch off all electronic devices, as the blue light emitted from them causes your levels of the hormone melatonin to drop off. This isn't good, as you need melatonin to be at its highest at night because it's what helps you fall asleep. What's more, it's now realised that the sleep hormone is produced in your gut as well as in your brain, and it's thought the gut version might work on a different cyclical rhythm from the melatonin made in your brain. Buy yourself an alarm clock and make your bedroom a 'no phone zone'.

- **Relax your face**
  Try some facial massage with a sleep-inducing oil – for instance, one infused with lavender or ylang-ylang. Using a few drops on cleansed skin, smooth it from the centre of your face outward, paying particular attention to the bony areas of your face, with long firm strokes over your cheekbones, across the tops of your eyebrows, in circular motions over your temples, and especially along your jawline by your back molars, which can hold a lot of tension.

- **Try a foot rub**
  Foot reflexology – pressing on certain points on the foot – can also help you unwind, especially pressing on the point linked to the diaphragm. First of all, squeeze your feet in your hands and gently knead them as you would dough. Doing this all over, from the heel up to the toes, will help relax as many internal organs as possible. Finish by pressing your thumb into the diaphragm or solar plexus point, which is just to the side of the ball of your foot, and down a bit – pretty much the dead-centre of the top half of your foot – and hold it for 10 seconds. This is a key stress-release trigger point.

- **Do forward bends**
  Yoga offers classic relaxation poses including the one we've probably all heard of – the child's pose. This involves kneeling close to the floor, relaxing your body over your thighs so your head touches the mat, with both arms down by your sides. Stay in this pose for as long as you like (from 20 seconds to 5 minutes), releasing tension from your body while breathing deeply and slowly – a very calming exercise for body and mind.

GOOD-GUT CHECKLIST

1. **Top up on magnesium**
   This multi-tasking mineral is a must-have, not only for keeping our blood pressure normal, our heart rhythm steady and our bones strong, but for relaxing muscles and helping us rest. Women over the age of 30 are advised to take 320mg a day, either as tablets or as powder dissolved in water. If you're pregnant, the levels rise to around 350mg a day.

2. **Boil your bones**
   Each time you have a roast chicken or cook a joint of meat, make sure you save the bones, then pop them in big pan or slow cooker to stew overnight. All the rich collagen will come out of the bone marrow and make a great stock, to be added to other recipes. Once strained, use as a basis for soups and have at least one portion per day during this week of healing and cleansing, to help nurture and 'seal' any leaky gut issues you may have.

3. **Love liquorice**
   Not only is the tea soothing, but another use of liquorice is to chew on the wild stem and use it as a way to clean your teeth and help combat gum disease.

4. **Soothe with aloe**
   Add a little aloe vera juice to your routine – try taking 50ml each morning before breakfast to coat your stomach in this naturally protective juice.

5. **Have a daily de-stress moment**
   It's so important to take at least five minutes out of your day to relax, breathe and reset. For example, if you've been hurrying about or been sitting at a desk for hours and find your shoulders are up around your ears, having a few moments to breathe deeply – extending the out-breaths so you're exhaling for longer – can really help you slow down and unwind, which is so important for a happy stomach. Try this before each meal, to assist digestion.

WEEK FIVE:
Balance

Perhaps it comes as a surprise to realise that our gut does so much more than just digest food and support our physical health – the fact is it also plays a major role in how we feel. This week we'll be considering how looking after our gut can help us achieve a healthy balance of wellbeing and actually make us feel happier.

From mindful eating to adding serotonin, dietary fibre and resistant starch to our meals, it's simply amazing how straightforward adjustments to good gut health can lift depression, and improve mood and mental health. What we eat – together with how and when we eat it, can make a real difference to mood and emotions. Personally, I feel more joyful when full of pre- and probiotics!

① Strengthen your serotonin

Our gut health has a huge influence on our moods and feelings – much greater than we might ever have thought. While depression used to be linked to low levels of serotonin in the brain – this being the neurotransmitter often credited with making us happy – it's now known that up to 90 per cent of this mood-regulating chemical is actually produced in the gut! There are specific cells in the intestines that produce serotonin and in 2015 researchers discovered that these cells depend on bacteria being present for them to do their job. Perhaps the reason most serotonin resides in the gut is because it's produced when we eat protein-rich foods containing the amino acid tryptophan. So for a genuinely feel-good food boost, tuck into the following tryptophan-rich foods:

Lean meat and seafood
Eat lean protein, which is a good source of tryptophan. The best poultry sources are turkey, duck and quail, while for seafood go for crab (especially Alaskan), prawns and lobster. Organic pork is also a good choice, as are game meats, the best of all being elk! All contain more than 500mg of tryptophan per 200-calorie serving (with elk at more than 700mg).

Go for green
No elk meat to hand? Spinach and watercress are also both rich in tryptophan – even more so than most of the meats mentioned above – though the best source of all is spirulina, the blue-green algae, which contains around the same amount of tryptophan as elk meat (and is slightly easier to get hold of).

Combine protein with carbs
While all proteins contain tryptophan, the best way to ensure full absorption is to eat carbs at the same time, according to the neuroscientist Alex Korb, who uses neuroscience to curb depression. For example, a 200-calorie serving of cooked oats – porridge, in fact – contains around 285mg of tryptophan, so porridge made from oats and milk is a good mood-boosting start to your morning.

Consider a supplement
Tryptophan converts to a substance called 5-HTP in our brain, which is why some may find taking 5-HTP supplements can help lift or ease low moods.

THE VAGUS NERVE AND WHY IT KEEPS US HAPPY

The vagus nerve has received remarkably little attention until very recently, when its role in sending messages between the gut and the brain became more fully understood. The longest nerve in our body, the vagus starts in the brain, then winds its way alongside the windpipe, before branching off into two main channels that pass through different organs and end up at the gut. The nerve is very complex, and it's still not known how all its functions fall into place. It's along this nerve that messages are sent from our gut up to our brain relating to how we're feeling and to what's going on down there. So those 'gut feelings' we get and butterflies in our stomach, which might make us feel nervous or sick, are all being transmitted upwards from our microbes to our brain.

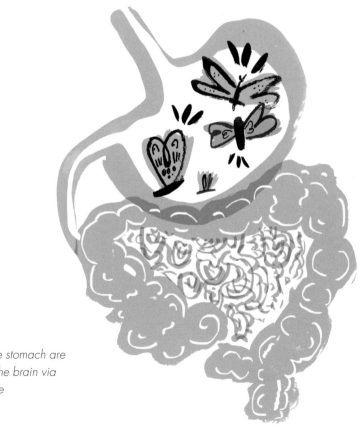

Butterflies in the stomach are transmitted to the brain via the vagus nerve

② Beat inflammation to reduce anxiety

Inflammation can be caused by stress, sugary and fried foods and hydrogenated fats, manmade chemicals, or dysbiosis in the gut that has built up over time – no chronic illness happens overnight. Eating an anti-inflammatory diet no doubt helps reduce inflammation in our gut, and that has a beneficial knock-on effect on our brain and nervous system. Low-grade gut inflammation has been found to cause anxiety-like behaviour in animals.

Certain substances found in food and drink can exacerbate anxiety, one of which is caffeine. It ramps up the production of the hormones adrenaline and cortisol, doubling it in the case of cortisol, which can add to any existing anxiety we may be feeling.

- **Continue to load up on the following**

  Berries: These vibrant little fruits help keep the brain healthy, thanks to their antioxidants. A long-term Harvard study, spread over 40 years, found that women who ate a handful of blueberries or a couple of handfuls of strawberries each week had better memories than those who hadn't. So once your gut is working well and absorbing more nutrients, try to make sure your weekly foods feature a few of these little brain-boosters.

  Nuts: When it comes to getting good fats into our diet, nuts are hugely helpful, especially the oilier varieties such as walnuts and macadamias. You may have been led to believe that nuts are bad because of their fat content, but it's all heart-healthy fats, so having a few a day will do us good, not harm. Remember, raw is best because removing the skins, as in blanching, also removes some of the antioxidant properties. Walnuts are superstars here, and the best brain-booster by far with their high concentrations of DHA, a type of Omega-3, which helps reduce age-related cognitive decline. Walnuts and their oil are also helpful in lowering our resting blood pressure, which is also good for the brain.

  Anti-inflammatory spices: Turmeric and ginger are two of the best anti-inflammatories in the spice world. To fully absorb all the healing properties of turmeric, add it to meals containing fat, such as coconut oil in a curry or avocado in a smoothie. Adding a pinch of black pepper also helps, as the piperine in it has recently been found to aid the absorption of turmeric's own healing substance, curcumin. Don't overheat (for instance with extended roasting or frying) as some studies suggest these spices' activity is reduced when cooked.

- **Limit your caffeine**

  Have just one cup a day, preferably in the morning – and try not to have it on an empty stomach.

- **Breathe to beat anxiety**

  When we're stressed or anxious, our breathing can become very shallow, to the point where it's all from our chest rather than originating deeper down. This can lead to pains in the chest that are coming from the muscles, not the heart, as well as feelings of hyperventilation, a more rapid heartbeat and maybe numbness in your extremities. The best thing to do is breathe deeply, but that's not always so easy to do if you're already in a panic! So, first make a long out-breath to make space for the in-breath. Do this with a deep sigh so as to relax your muscles; hold for a few counts. Then, with mouth closed, slowly breathe in through your nose, feeling your stomach push out as you do so. Once your stomach is as large as it will go, let it go. Avoid bringing your chest into the breath – the point is to keep it down low to relax and de-stress you.

③ Eat mindfully

As well as eating a healthy diet and taking supplements, one of the easiest ways to give our gut a chance to do its jobs effectively is to slow down and savour our meals. We've all been guilty of tapping away on our phones or iPads while gulping down a snack, but this makes it harder for our gut to digest, which can lead to poor nutrient absorption and indigestion. Chewing slowly and mindfully, enjoying our food and taking our time, helps our body get into the rest-and-digest mode as opposed to the fight-or-flight response.

- At all mealtimes sit down at a table and, before you begin eating, take a few long, deep breaths to calm your heart rate. The more relaxed you can be, the better, as stress negatively affects digestion.

- Focus all of your attention on your food: how does it look, smell and feel in your mouth? Chew slowly too; the more times the better (25 times before you swallow is a good guideline). This not only helps you slow down but will mean your stomach has less work to do when the food arrives.

- The more stressed or anxious you are, the more likely you'll want to grab something sugary, so try keeping some healthy high-fat snacks to hand such as nuts, a small chunk of unpasteurised cheese with oatcakes, or some hummus and crudités.

- Take a good multi-strain probiotic daily and/ or add sauerkraut or kimchi to dishes to help boost their good-bacteria content, as diversity in the gut means you're likely to feel happier. You'll find my favourite recipes for these in Part Two.

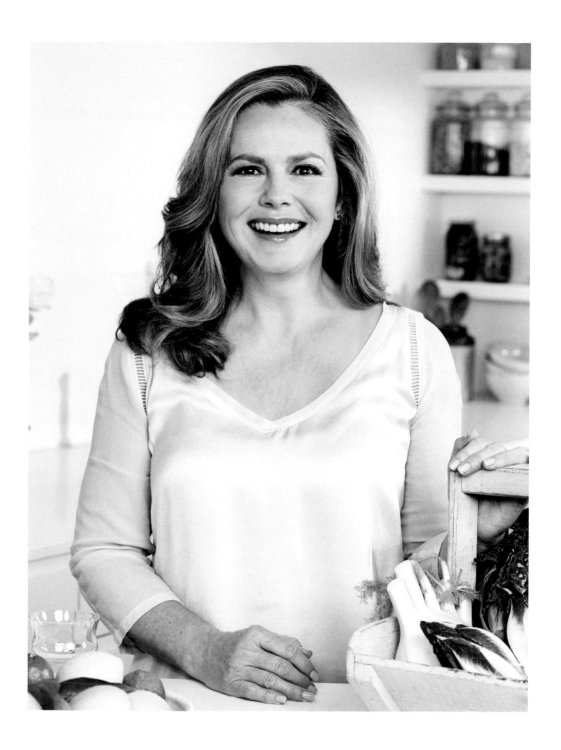

④ Balance your blood sugar

Sugar, as we've seen, is also a culprit when it comes to poor gut health and, as a consequence, low mood. A hit of refined sugar causes our blood sugar to rise rapidly – which is then followed by a slump in energy and a feeling of lethargy, and all because our hormones have gone haywire. 'People so often just think about diabetes or obesity when they hear the term blood sugar, but it's intrinsically linked to mood as well,' says Dr Rangan Chatterjee, an NHS GP and self-confessed 'real-food junkie'. This is because it disrupts our hormones, which normally all work together.

'No hormone works in isolation. When, two hours after eating a huge sugary meal, you have a crash in blood sugar, it's not only that your insulin plummets, but cortisol and adrenaline, two hormones associated with stress, sky-rocket,' he says. 'This puts your body into the "fight-or-flight" mode, which pushes you into a stressed state. Stabilising your blood sugar therefore has a positive effect on adrenaline and cortisol levels.'

Balancing blood sugar helps alleviate not only everyday anxiety but also panic attacks, if you're prone to them. So, it's not only wise to moderate our sugar intake but, if we do eat it, to have it along with other foods such as protein and vegetables to mitigate the effects.

- **Opt for slow-release carbs**
  Choose brown rice and pseudo-grains such as quinoa and buckwheat. If you really fancy a handful of potato crisps, eat them with a gut-healing avocado dip, or a healthy fat-filled tahini-based hummus (only if your digestion can tolerate chickpeas). But to really avoid sugar spikes and bring down your blood sugar levels, you're best off eating a largely Paleo (that is, Paleolithic, or caveman) type diet of meat, vegetables and few, if any, carbs – at least for a month or so.

- **Eat protein with your carbs**
  Combining sweet or carb-rich foods with protein helps lessen the blood sugar spike. Eat chicken, fish or eggs with rice or potatoes, and have meat or fish with pasta. A good way to get a nice balance of flavours, including a little hit of sweetness, is to add dried fruits to a savoury dish, such as apricots in a lamb tagine. Or eat fruits with nuts and some cheese. This is preferable to eating a handful of dried fruit on its own, as the effect on blood sugar is pretty much the same as munching sugar cubes.

- **Try a fat-filled sweet treat**
  If you're craving chocolate, forgo the bars in the supermarket – even the 70 per cent cocoa ones often have sugar as their second ingredient – and instead buy a tub of raw cacao. Put a tablespoon or two, depending on how chocolatey you want it, into 500ml of almond milk along with a tablespoon of coconut oil, or half an avocado. Blitz this up and enjoy a creamy chocolate drink – or you can gently heat it up as a warming treat during the day instead of coffee.

⑤ Boost our fibre intake

By far one of the unsung heroes of the food world, probably because it's not 'sexy' like sweet- or fat-filled foods, is fibre. Yet we absolutely need fibre to stay healthy. Some types are fermented in our lower intestine, the colon, by all those good bugs that use it for energy and to create other healthy by-products. So although it's currently fashionable to eat a diet high in protein and fat, please don't cut out fibre – it's crucial for keeping all that protein moving along our intestines. We're meant to consume around 30g of fibre a day but this is rarely achieved in a standard Western diet.

There are three main types of fibre found in food – soluble and insoluble, and resistant starches:

Soluble fibre

Also known as fermentable fibre, this creates a gel-like texture when it mixes with liquid in our GI tract. It helps slow down digestion and makes us feel fuller for longer. What's more, soluble fibre attaches itself to cholesterol particles in the gut, taking them with it and thereby reducing overall cholesterol levels as well as the risk of heart disease. Find it in oats, barley and rye, bananas, apples, beans and other pulses, and root vegetables such as carrots and potatoes.

Insoluble fibre

This fibre doesn't dissolve, so if you're suffering from constipation, it will help push things along nicely. It helps stools stay soft yet bulky, so they can easily transit the colon. Add more of it to your diet in the form of oats, wholegrains, raw fruits and vegetables, potatoes with their skin on, brown rice, wheat bran, golden linseed, nuts, seeds and, of course, prunes, which are perhaps the ultimate unblocker. Although we need it in our diets, those with IBS or otherwise sensitive stomachs can get bloated from eating too much insoluble fibre. Try the following preparation tips to minimise any negative impact:

1. Make soups, sauces and dips from fruit and vegetables instead of eating them whole or raw.

2. Blend fresh fruit into a smoothie and have it after a breakfast of porridge.

3. Add lentils or other pulses to sauces or soups or use them in dips, to make them easier to digest.

4. Eat raw fruit at the beginning of a meal instead of at the end so that it has time to digest properly. Fruit only takes around 30 minutes to be digested, whereas protein takes a few hours. This means a fruit salad for dessert can sit waiting to be digested, giving it the chance to ferment and lead to that dreaded bloating feeling.

5. If you're suffering from a bout of diarrhoea try removing the skins of fruits and vegetables, as that's where more of the insoluble kind of fibre is found.

H$_2$0

Make sure you drink plenty of water as increased fibre can cause constipation, the very thing we're seeking to banish. If you don't like drinking lots of plain water, you can always sweeten it with one of the recipes in Part Two of this book – just avoid artificially sweetened waters, as the synthetic chemicals in these can upset the balance of our microbiome.

I've used a water filter jug for decades as I think it's the easiest and cheapest way to get purer, fresher-tasting water for cooking and drinking. A simple filter screens out the chlorine routinely added to mains water and which kills off our beneficial bacteria. Drinking weak solutions of chlorine is not a great idea when we're trying to preserve our microflora.

Resistant starches

Most carbohydrates contain 'resistant starches', which are resistant to digestion, hence their name. You find them in green bananas, legumes and cashew nuts, as well as in cooked then cooled potatoes and rice. They've been shown to improve insulin sensitivity (helpful for diabetes), lower blood sugar levels, reduce appetite and benefit digestion. Try the following

1. Eat cold potatoes
   'These become a useful source of prebiotics and help create a platform for healthy gut bacteria to grow,' says Sue Davis, a naturopath and Western medical herbalist. 'The cooling process creates resistant starch, which acts like dietary fibre so it is beneficial for bowel health. But I would recommend removing the skins if suffering from IBS as these will be harder to break down,' says Sue, who doesn't advise reheating cold potatoes as once reheated they can cause indigestion if they have been stored or reheated incorrectly. 'Plus, reheating will cause a large percentage of the vitamin C content to be lost.' A better idea would be to make a potato salad with some digestion-boosting herbs and probiotic-rich unpasteurised cheese

2. Eat sushi
   Cooked sushi rice is also a form of resistant starch, so if you're generally eating low carbs, you could have a couple of portions of nigiri-style sushi each week.

GOOD-GUT CHECKLIST

1. **Fill your plate with fibre**
   To get a good mixture of the soluble and insoluble varieties, make sure you include plenty of leafy and root vegetables, pulses, oats and other grains in your diet each day – in fact, the bulk of our meals should consist of fibrous foods.

2. **Relax before eating**
   Make more time to slow down and savour your meals. Eating on the go means you're less likely to produce enough digestive juices needed for optimum digestion. Before each meal, sit comfortably, still and quietly, then take five long, deep breaths to calm your body and mind.

3. **Eat anti-inflammatory food**
   Do both your head and gut brains a favour and stick to fresh unprocessed foods such as leafy greens and healthy fats, and limit any refined sugars and carbs. If you're not a veggie fan, try blitzing them into a soup, or try a smoothie along with some fruit – and your kefir or kombucha – so as to still get your quota for the day.

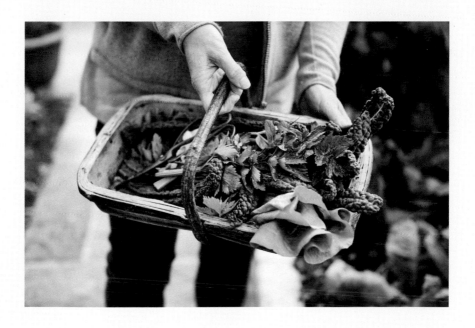

WEEK SIX:
Maintenance and Radiance

After five weeks of healthily detoxing and cleansing your system, as well as repopulating your gut with both flora-friendly prebiotics and perhaps probiotic supplements, now's the time to move on to discover how to maintain your new-found inner health and outer radiance by eating foods your good bugs will just love you for.

Most cultures around the world have their own favourite form of fermented foods as part of their national cuisine, from German sauerkraut to French crème fraîche, Korean kimchi, Japanese miso, Greek yoghurt and Polish kvass. Consuming some fermented or 'cultured' foods and drinks each day is a good habit to get into. Some of these strange-sounding foods are an acquired taste, often slightly sour or fizzy, but after a short while you may find they become more pleasantly 'addictive' – almost as if your body's microbial crowd starts crying out for more.

⓵ Fermenting

Fermented foods and drinks are having their moment in the wellbeing world and it's all do to with our new best friends – bacteria.

Fermentation occurs in the absence of oxygen, allowing natural bacteria to proliferate. The bacteria feed on the sugars in foods, thereby dramatically reducing the foods' sugar content to the point where even diabetics are able to consume them. In fact, these foods are teeming with so many beneficial microbes that they've been shown to improve microbial diversity in our gut as well as balancing our metabolism to keep us slim by curbing our sugar cravings. The fibres in cultured or fermented vegetables also help feed beneficial gut bacteria.

With so many benefits, it's no wonder these 'ancient' foods are making a comeback. Fermented foods are definitely an acquired taste – often quite tangy, tart or sharp. But they add a nice balance to dishes that might otherwise be too sweet or even bland. If you're new to fermented foods, introduce them gradually. We've waited until Week Six to focus on them because it's best first to kill off any yeast infections or suspected parasites you may be harbouring. In some instances, fermented foods can feed the bad yeasts – the last thing you need. They may take a bit of getting used to, but trust me on this one, you'll soon grow to love them and may even develop a healthy addiction to their tangy tastes. One word of caution here: fermented foods and drinks can be a trigger for some who get migraine headaches.

Once you incorporate these newcomers into your daily diet, your digestion will soon improve and you'll have healthier-looking skin and be brimming with energy and vitality!

Fermented friends

Sauerkraut

Sauerkraut is usually made just from cabbage but you can make it with pretty much any other vegetables in the mix. In a simpler form it has been around for more than 3,000 years and was one of the commonest ways of preserving cabbage. Making your own is much better than buying pre-packaged pasteurised sauerkraut, devoid of all the good bacteria and enzymes (see my recipe on page 108). As with cultured dairy products, the fermentation process involved in making sauerkraut produces plenty of the beneficial bacteria linked to improvements in immunity, brain health, digestion and endocrine function. And we need only to add a few forkfuls to meals each day to get the benefits.

Kvass

Traditionally made with fermented barley or sourdough rye bread and popular in countries such as Poland, kvass is now becoming a big thing in the world of fermented drinks (see page 238). While it's considered non-alcoholic it does contain a tiny amount, though usually less than 1 per cent, but it gets more alcoholic the longer you let it ferment, of course. Depending on what you use to make it, it can have a variety of flavours such as fruits and herbs, although overall it has an earthy taste. It's often made with beetroots, a good blood nourisher that improves stamina and helps us stay energised. Kvass contains helpful amounts of trace minerals and important vitamins including vitamin B12 as well as manganese, and it's a great liver detoxifier. Some also take it as a digestive tonic.

Kombucha

Pronounced kom-boo-cha, this fermented drink has had a recent boost in popularity, although I've been making it for at least twenty years. It's made by putting what they call a 'kombucha baby' or 'scoby' (which stands for Symbiotic Culture Of Bacteria and Yeast) into hot water, with sugar and green or black teabags, and letting it ferment. The 'kombucha baby' is aptly named as it looks embryonic and slimy – but what it lacks in looks it makes up for in health benefits! The tea is reputed to help our body build strong defences against bad bugs and infections. It can taste quite sour, though with a slightly fizzy sweetness, and is perfect mixed with sparkling apple juice or other juices. You can also ferment it for longer so it turns into vinegar, which can be used for pickling and preserving other foods. I chill my kombucha drink and serve it in wineglasses on the days I'm not drinking alcohol. Delicious (see my recipe on page 104).

Kimchi

This fermented dish native to Korea is made of fermented cabbage and sometimes radishes, as well as garlic, salt, vinegar, chilli peppers and spices – making it a pretty potent side dish or salsa. The Koreans love it and eat it with almost every meal. It's said to be the reason there's a very low incidence of obesity in the country, thanks to its high fibre content and raft of probiotics, namely ones belonging to the *Lactobacillus* group which are good for digestion, as we've seen. It's also packed with vitamins B and C and beta-carotene, which may be easier for our body to absorb here, thanks to the good bacteria present. As with sauerkraut, just a small serving a day is plenty – large amounts can cause bloating. Try my recipe on page 110.

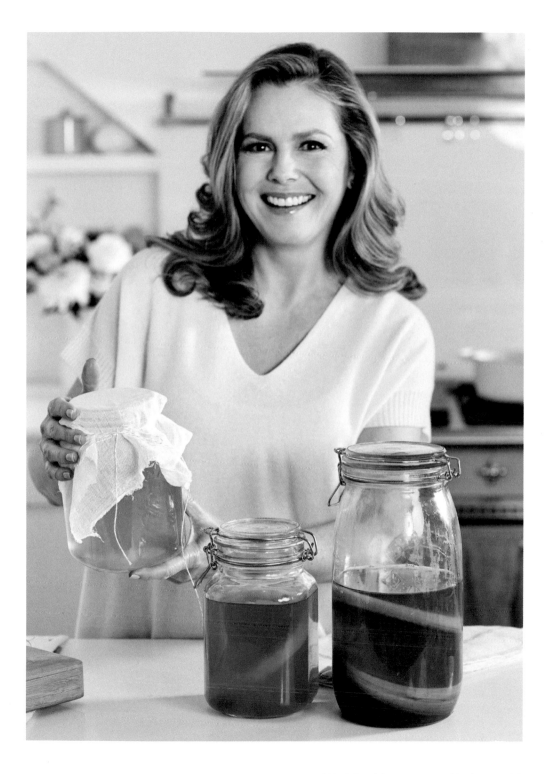

Ginger ale

The original ginger ale – unlike the mass-produced extremely sugary versions sold in bottles and cans – comes from another live yeast/bacterial culture. The culture – called a 'ginger bug' – divides and grows in the same way as others do and some can be hundreds of years old. When added to a solution of water, sugar and ginger powder, it's easy to make your own healthily probiotic-packed drink. As with kombucha, the sugar in the water mostly gets eaten up during the fermentation process, so don't be put off by the amount used.

Make your own ginger ale

MAKES ABOUT 2 LITRES
PREP: 10 MINUTES, PLUS FERMENTING TIME (UP TO ABOUT 11 DAYS)

For the ginger bug:
5cm piece fresh ginger, peeled and finely sliced
110g granulated sugar
500ml filtered water

For the ginger ale:
1.6 litres filtered water
5cm piece fresh ginger, peeled and minced
100g granulated sugar
Juice of 1 lemon or lime
Pinch sea salt

Equipment: A 2-litre sterilised sealable jar

- First make the ginger bug. Put all but 1 tbsp of the ginger in the jar, tip in 100g of the sugar and pour in the water. Stir with a wooden spoon, seal and put to one side – in the kitchen is fine.

- The next day add 1 tbsp of finely sliced ginger and the remaining granulated sugar, then stir again with the wooden spoon. It should start to bubble within 8 days. When this happens it's ready for the next stage.

- For the ginger ale add 600ml of the water to a saucepan along with the fresh ginger and the sugar and bring to the boil. Simmer for a few minutes until the sugar dissolves. Remove from the heat and pour in the remaining water. Leave it to cool completely, then add the lemon or lime juice and pour in the ginger bug that you've prepared.

- Pour all the mixture back into the jar and seal. Leave for 2–3 days – it will be OK in the kitchen and should soon start to carbonate and ferment. Strain into a sterilised bottle or jar and keep in the fridge until ready to use. You may need to strain it again before drinking.

Kefir

Kefir too is a fermented drink, most often made from cow's milk but it can also be made with coconut milk, coconut water or any other nut 'milks'. It's probably up there at the top of my list for probiotic foods, as it contains such a large diversity of probiotic strains. It's also a good store-cupboard staple because you can use kefir in a number of ways – for example, as a base for smoothies or as a 'milk' on cereals and in desserts. Because it does tend to have the smell and consistency of sour milk, especially if you let if ferment more than a couple of days (the longer you leave it, the thicker and creamier it gets), you might want to add fruit or raw honey to sweeten. Make sure your family know not to throw it out – it hasn't gone off, it's meant to smell like that!

Milk

There's much debate as to whether or not we should drink cow's milk. I believe cow's milk can be good for us when it's in its natural form – that is, when it comes from organically raised, grass-fed cows that have not been routinely treated with antibiotics for mastitis or given grain feed they normally wouldn't eat. I buy local milk from grass-grazed cows (I especially like organic unhomogenised whole milk from Ayreshire cows).

You may like to check out raw milk – it won't have been pasteurised (heat-treated). Raw milk contains more vitamins, minerals, enzymes and fatty acids (and natural probiotics) than pasteurised. Pasteurisation was introduced to protect the public from tuberculosis in the 1950s and was highly effective at reducing the death toll from this infectious disease. However, raw-milk devotees now argue that modern hygiene methods and home refrigeration make raw milk safe to drink, especially in areas where there's no bovine TB. Either way, raw milk can only legally be sold direct from the farmer, which these days can include vending machines.

Drinking milk is a personal preference, but if you want to avoid animal milk altogether or are lactose-intolerant, alternatives abound – from coconut to almond, cashew, soya, oat, rice milks and more. These don't have the same 'live' benefits of dairy milk, nor the valuable vitamin D or calcium content so helpful for strong, healthy bones. But they are still good to make kefir from if you have a starter culture to get things going.

Sourdough

Now, you may be thinking, 'But bread makes me bloat, so how can it be that good?' Well, a common reason why most commercially produced loaves lead to tummy trouble is to do with the presence of a substance called phytic acid. All grains and seeds contain phytic acid to protect them and keep their inner nutrients intact. So although many health experts say grains are good for us because they contain vitamins and minerals – which is correct – we can't easily access those health-boosting nutrients such as calcium, magnesium, iron and zinc because they're 'locked in' by the phytic acid. And phytic acid irritates the stomach lining.

However, there's a type of bread that's much easier to digest: sourdough. The wild yeast and *Lactobacillus* bacteria contained within the leaven help to predigest the flour and release the nutrients, while neutralising the gut-irritating phytic acid. The long, slow fermentation is also what gives sourdough such a great taste. So if you've been avoiding bread for fear of bloating, give sourdough a try (see page 100).

② Omega-3s

The essential fatty acid called Omega-3 is vital for good gut health as well as brain health – it keeps not only our intestines healthy but our brain cells too, staving off degenerative diseases. Our brain is around 60 per cent fat, the cell walls of which are made of Omega-3 – or at least a healthy brain should be. Upping our Omega-3 levels is helpful for health and vitality at all ages and stages of our life, especially for developing young brains.

OPTIMUM OMEGAS

- **Eat at least two portions of oily fish a week**
  This takes in salmon, fresh tuna, mackerel, sardines and herring, including the skins as that's where the most Omega-3 is found. The smaller ones such as sardines and mackerel will be less likely to contain a build-up of heavy metals, unlike the larger fish tuna and swordfish, which is also better for our brain in the long run.

- **Include flax seeds**
  Vegetarians, vegans and meat-eaters alike can use flax seeds, either ground up as meal or as the extracted oil, although flax seeds provide Omega-3 only in the form of alpha-linolenic acid (ALA), which is nowhere near as effective as the DHA and EPA Omega fats found in fish. The body needs to convert ALA into EPA to be effective.

- **Consider supplementing with algae oil**
  The reason fish are such good sources of DHA and EPA is actually because of their algae-rich diet, so why not go straight to the source? There are plenty of vegetarian and vegan Omega-3 brands.

3 Soothe your gut with stomach yoga

You may be familiar with the fabulous de-stressing effects of yoga. A grounding hatha yoga class or a deeply relaxing yin yoga session is helpful for both soothing the mind and calming the body – and especially for helping us to switch from fight-or-flight to rest-and-digest mode. Most types of yoga will be good for our whole body, but did you know there's a type designed specifically for helping us digest and beat bloating? Not only will you get a moment to yourself to calm the mind, you'll be improving the health of your 'second brain' too.

The following moves are from Elena Voyce, founder of Teach Yoga (teachyoga.com) and a practitioner for the past twenty or more years. She has created these exercises to help encourage movement and relaxation in the digestive organs, to ease cramping and constipation and reduce abdominal tension.

TRY TONGUE-PULLING TO REDUCE TENSION

Your tongue can affect what's going on lower down in your digestive system if it's tense or tight, perhaps through stress. This inhibits the production of saliva and the enzymes needed to digest food. Manipulating your tongue by gently pulling on it can help loosen it to aid digestion.

1. Hold your tongue with a clean cloth so it doesn't slip.

2. Wiggle it up, down and side to side a few times, holding it in each direction for a few seconds each. This helps reduce any tightness in the back of your throat and mouth.

USE A BLOCK TO HELP UNBLOCK!

You can help relieve constipation by lying on top of a rolled-up towel or yoga block. This compresses your digestive organs to encourage peristalsis, which is the action of your stools being moved along by the muscles in the large intestine.

1. With either a soft yoga block or a rolled-up towel placed along the centre of your stomach, from rib cage down to pubic bone, lie face down on a mat and breathe deeply for around 10 breaths. You may feel uncomfortable at first, but try to relax and soften your body around the object.

2. Come up slowly, placing your hands by your shoulders to push yourself up.

ROTATE TO RELIEVE BACK TENSION

Sometimes sluggish digestion is caused by tightness in your back. This move can help you release any tension there.

1. Lie on the floor facing down, feet together, with your knees and arms bent at right angles, head facing to the left.

2. Take a nice deep breath in; as you exhale, twist your pelvis and legs to the right. On the next inhale, bring your lower body back again. Do this five times before repeating on the other side, head facing to the right this time.

3. Finish off, with your lower body rotated, by pushing up through your hands to lift your upper body off the ground. Lower and raise your upper body like this five times on each side.

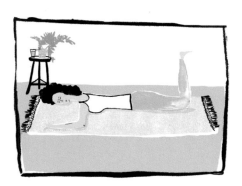

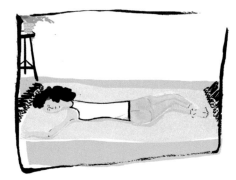

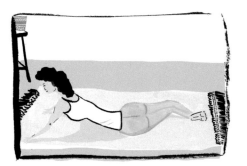

TRY FORWARD BENDS TO EASE HEARTBURN

People with acid reflux, stomach acidity or heartburn should avoid doing the yoga downward-facing dog pose as it can exacerbate the problem. Instead, try this simple move using a chair. It gives you all the same benefits but without the upper-body pressure that comes from doing a full downward dog.

1. Stand about a metre in front of a stable chair or table, and reach your arms out onto it so your body forms a right angle, head looking up.

2. Now, lower your head as you exhale, then lift it again on the inhale. Do this nodding movement five times to promote a stretch along your back.

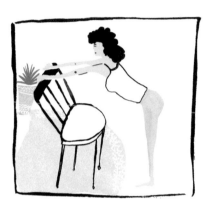 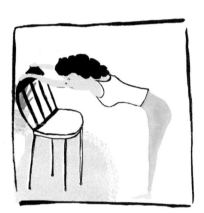

USE SOOTHING CIRCLES TO BEAT THE BLOAT

Massaging your digestive organs by applying firm (but not painful) pressure can help reduce acidity and relieve bloating and cramping.

1. Start with your hands on the right side of your tummy, midway between your hip and lower rib. Move them in circles, clockwise, seven times. This helps both stimulate and soothe your large intestine.

2. Then make smaller circles in the same direction around the navel a couple of times to do the same for your small intestine.

④ Sprout your grains

Nuts and seeds can also be difficult for some of us to break down. If in the past you've avoided nuts because they give you tummy trouble, you might want to experiment with soaking them overnight. The same with seeds. Soaking softens the tough outer layer and reduces the phytate (or phytic acid) content, the part that makes them indigestible. Just put them in a bowl, cover them with water and leave overnight, then rinse in the morning before using. To make them even easier to digest, blitz up in smoothies so you not only get all the antioxidants of the fruit and veg, you also get a dose of healthy fats to reduce the GI effects on your blood sugar.

Whether or not you have trouble digesting grains you might want to consider sprouting them – that is, soaking them and allowing them to germinate. The nutritional benefits include up to 75 per cent fewer carbohydrates in the form of starch than wholegrains, plus more protein. They also help our gut absorb more nutrients from other foods eaten at the same time. Sprouted grains are less gas-producing, too, which is good news for anyone with IBS.

- **Start sprouting!**
  Depending on the type of grain, soak them either overnight or for a few hours in some cases, then leave them, damp, in a jar covered with a muslin cloth or in a specially designed sprouting tray (available online). Soak the grains or seeds – you can use any as long as they haven't been processed (that is, they must be in their raw form) – in clean water overnight, then put them into the jar or sprouter.

- **Rinse the grains every 12 hours in a sieve, then put them back**
  This is to keep them clean. They should sprout – little shoots will appear – in a couple of days. Rinse, dry, then refrigerate and eat

  them within a few days. If you don't fancy making your own, supermarkets are now selling pre-sprouted legumes and seeds, so look out for them in the fresh-produce aisles. Always rinse well before use and check their use-by date.

- **A safety note**
  Use clean, fresh water because on the odd occasion sprouts can become contaminated with bad bacteria (though usually only if they're left in the same water for too long). For this reason, official guidelines say pregnant women, the elderly and anyone with a compromised immune system should avoid them.

⑤ Herbal healers

As we've seen, nature provides us with an array of foods to keep our tummies happy, and herbs are yet another healing powerhouse in our good-gut toolkit. One of my favourite at-home rituals is to make tasty teas containing fresh or dried herbs, many of which can also help soothe an upset stomach and digestive disorders.

Fennel

Such a versatile digestive aid, the fennel bulb is a good source of fibre to help reduce our cholesterol levels and cleanse the colon. The seeds of the fennel plant are particularly effective when made into a tea, and are popular in Ayurvedic medicine and in plenty of herbal digestion products. The essential oil has been found to have a relaxing effect and can reduce muscle spasms in the gut.

Make your own liquorice and peppermint tea

Peppermint is one of our best-known digestion-boosting herbs and when added to liquorice root, which can help heal leaky gut, this makes for a powerful tummy-soothing tea.

Serves 2

6cm piece liquorice root
1 tsp dried peppermint leaves

1 cardamom pod, seeds only
400ml hot filtered water (not boiling)

Put the liquorice root, peppermint leaves and cardamom seeds into a small teapot. Pour over the water and leave to steep for 5 minutes, then strain, to serve.

Mint

Most varieties of mint, such as peppermint and spearmint, help calm the digestive system, hence its popularity over millennia as a remedy for indigestion. Peppermint also helps relieve gas and bloating, and taking peppermint oil capsules can be an effective treatment for IBS.

Make a soothing cup of tea, with fresh mint leaves if available – the smell is truly fabulous – or use a mint teabag. Look for tea in unbleached teabags, as the bright-white bleached variety may be made from material dipped in chlorine (a potent good-bug killer).

Making your own mint tea with freshly picked leaves is simply the best. Just pour hot water (not boiling, as this scalds the leaves) over a handful of fresh mint in a mug or teapot, steep for 3–4 minutes, then pour through a strainer (though the leaves are likely to stay in the spout, especially if they're still on the stalk).

- **Make a minty mocktail**
  Try adding mint leaves with some fresh lemon juice to your kombucha recipe, for a refreshing summer nojito.

- **Improve your digestion of fruit**
  Although fruit is best eaten on its own as it passes through our system faster than other foods, if you do end up having it for pudding, add a sprinkling of mint leaves to help the digestion process.

- **Try natural mint choc-tips!**
  If you're craving something sweet, try using chocolate mint (a plant variety) as a tisane instead of regular mint leaves. The leaves are slightly smaller and brown underneath – and they really do smell of chocolate!

- **Retain the flavour**
  When cooking with mint, use a very sharp knife, as a blunt one can blacken and bruise the leaves and may reduce their potency.

Nettle

These weeds may annoy us outdoors, but don't be too quick to dig them up and throw them on the compost heap – instead, try letting a small patch grow so you have at your fingertips your own fresh nettles to make a gut-healing tea. Because of its antihistamine and anti-inflammatory properties, nettle can also be used to alleviate eczema, either internally to soothe the itch from within or used in a topical cream – just don't rub the leaves on your skin.

Triphala

Traditionally used as a bowel tonic, this natural blend is often prescribed as a mild laxative. But while its laxative qualities are most widely known, the other benefits of this trio of herbs are perhaps even more noteworthy. Triphala means 'three fruits', and it comprises the fruits of the Indian plants amalaki, haritaki and bibhitaki. Amalaki is shown to help lower our cholesterol and is loaded with vitamin C, as well as helping prevent diarrhoea; haritaki is anti-inflammatory, while bibhitaki detoxifies the blood and the fatty tissue of the body. Together these three powerful, cleansing herbs encourage proper elimination, which is especially good for those with constipation. You'll find triphala as a powder or as capsules, and it's a popular supplement in Ayurvedic medicine.

A SAFETY NOTE: Possible side effects are similar to those caused by high-fibre foods or supplements, such as loose stools, gas and bloating. It is not advised during pregnancy.

So when it comes to supporting our gut, strengthening and balancing our immune system, and basically giving our insides the best chance to stay healthy, the following checklist will keep us on the right path.

GOOD-GUT CHECKLIST

1. **Try yoga**
   While you won't want to be bending and stretching right after a meal, if you're still feeling bloated an hour or so later try massaging your tummy as in the digestion yoga on page 87. You can also try the belly rub while in the bath, or use some massage oil, both of which make it easier to glide your fingers over your skin

2. **Improve the digestibility of carbs by sprouting your own**
   Experiment with sprouting a few grains, seeds and legumes to see whether it helps reduce any bloating you might have. Eating these super-sprouts helps increase the amounts of food we're able to absorb, leading to faster digestion and more energy. Add a few sprouted seeds to your breakfast, and some sprouted pulses to salads or roasted veggies.

3. **Grow herbs**
   Using herbs regularly in cooking, especially fennel and mint, can help our digestive tract stay healthy. Why not grow some mint on a windowsill? It's so easy to pick up a pot from the supermarket. Use it to make tea to drink after meals.

4. **Feast on fermented foods**
   Add a spoonful of sauerkraut or kimchi to your lunch or supper. A tablespoonful totally transforms a plain baked potato and adds a taste sensation to salads.

Every day:

- First thing: drink warm water with a little lemon juice squeezed into it to alkalise your gut. Or juice celery and try that neat or mixed with a little water too.

- Take a multi-strain, multibillion-microbe probiotic, ideally on an empty stomach (look for one with at least eight different strains).

- Have a few spoonfuls of fermented vegetables, such as sauerkraut or kimchi, perhaps with lunch or supper.

- Slow down when you eat. Take 10 slow, deep breaths before starting each meal and chew mindfully. Try not to eat on the go, standing up or under stress.

- Exercise, even if it's just a daily walk. This not only keeps your gut moving but also helps you relax. Do some digestion yoga stretches too.

- Try 5–10 minutes of meditation at the beginning and/or end of your day. This helps calm both brain and gut.

Every week:

- Make a fresh kombucha brew and find a friend to donate your spare scoby to! It's good to share knowledge and wellbeing wisdom here.

- Encourage friends and family out into the fresh air with some brisk Nordic or power walking, or organise a group run if that's more your thing, and allow the impact to gently stimulate your digestive system.

Every month:

- Try a juice-only day when you drink just pure vegetable juices sweetened with a little fruit. This will give your GI tract an opportunity to rest and regenerate. Top up with plenty of pure filtered water.

Every 3 months:

- Consider a bentonite clay or psyllium cleanse, especially if you're aware your gut health has been compromised over the years.

- Give yourself a gut-healing weekend. Simply plan a quiet 24 or 48 hours at home with minimum outside disturbances, and schedule some light eating, juicing, walking, magnesium baths and general rest and relaxation. Book the time into your diary and – make it happen!

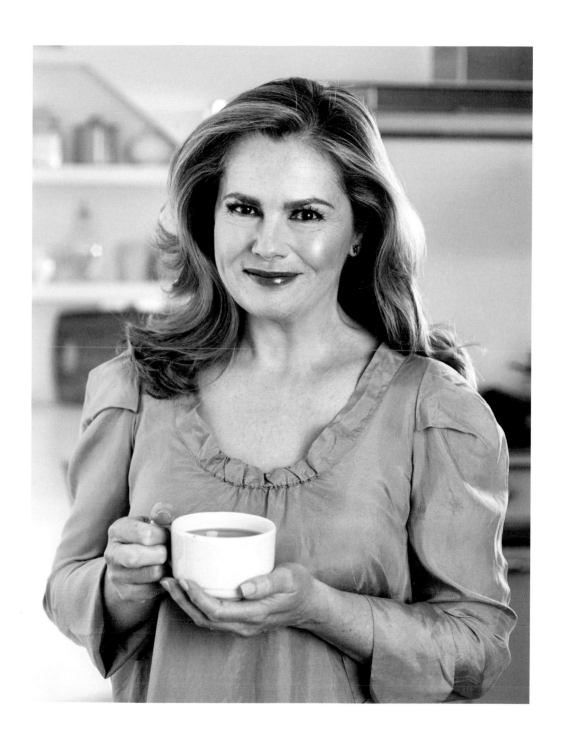

PART TWO: RECIPES

Getting Started

Making your own super-healthy, probiotic, gut-healing foods is easier than you might think and it's worth investing in a few key bits of kit to get started. See my equipment list below and I've also included stockists and helpful websites at the back of this book (see page 246).

Equipment checklist:

SAUERKRAUT: Basic mason or Kilner jars work well, but you'll also find purpose-made jars that contain a pounder to tamp down the veggies, weights to keep everything tightly packed and special air-lock lids to keep the air out.

KIMCHI: Use the same kind of jars as for sauerkraut. You'll also need a really large bowl for mixing up the ingredients. Food preparation gloves are also useful.

KEFIR: A couple of large jars and a few muslin cloths are really all the kit you need here. It's always good to have a couple so that when one jar starts to get low, you can use a few spoonfuls of the kefir to start off another jar, meaning you don't always need to start with fresh grains each time. Elastic bands are useful for holding the muslin cloths in place and sticky labels help keep track of how long things have been fermenting. Any cultured product needs a starter culture to get going, so you'll need to buy a pack of kefir starter grains (freeze-dried or fresh bacteria) to make your first batch. Many kefir aficionados like to use fresh live grains as they contain more beneficial bacteria, (up to fifty strains of yeasts and bacteria), particularly *Lactobacillus*. Also, the freeze-dried versions do have a shelf life so they lose potency over time. But live kefir grains or, say, a sourdough starter, can last indefinitely if cared for correctly.

SOURDOUGH BREAD: This also needs a starter culture, which you can make yourself (see page 100). You might also want to invest in a proofing basket, similar to the rattan or wicker baskets used by bakers. This will help shape the loaf during its final rise before you put it into the oven. Or use a colander or bowl lined with a tea towel sprinkled with flour to prevent the dough sticking.

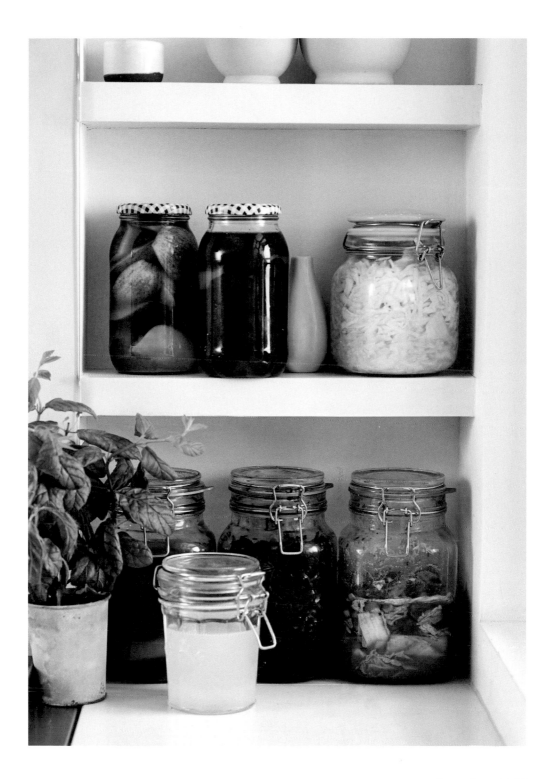

Spelt Sourdough
STEP BY STEP

If you've ever fancied making your own artisan sourdough bread, here's my perfect starter recipe. Few things beat the smell of freshly baked bread – it's homely, inviting and comforting. And if bread makes you feel bloated, this sourdough loaf could be just what you need to satisfy a carb craving without messing with your microbiome. Sourdough is naturally fermented, meaning the tough outer shell of the grain is broken down before we eat it. This makes it a lot easier to absorb, and gentler on our gut. Try a slice or two for breakfast, warmed and served with melted butter (organic and grass-fed, if you can), for a healthy dose of butyrate to boost your good-gut bugs.

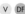 **V DF MAKES 2 MEDIUM-SIZED LOAVES**
TAKES 50 MINUTES PLUS FERMENTING TIME (THIS CAN BE UP TO 2 WEEKS)   192 calories (per slice)

For the starter:
130g white spelt flour
40g wholemeal spelt flour
200ml tepid water
Note: You will need more of each to 'feed'
    the starter

For the dough:
140g starter

250ml water
320g white spelt flour, sieved, plus some for
    dusting
160g wholemeal spelt flour
Pinch sea salt
Drizzle of extra virgin olive oil

Equipment: 2 proving baskets dusted with flour
    (optional)

To make the starter

- Add the flours and water to a glass bowl or container and combine, cover with a piece of cloth or muslin and set aside in the kitchen at room temperature (around 20°C).

- The starter should begin to bubble slightly the next day. Use a quarter of your starter and combine with a further 100g white spelt flour, 20g wholemeal and 100ml water. Stir and add a little more water if it looks dry. It should look similar to batter before you feed it and should increase in size just after you have fed it. Cover again and set aside in the kitchen.

- Repeat this process every day, taking a quarter of the mixture, feeding it and leaving it to rest at room temperature. At around 5–9 days it should start to smell a little acidic and be filled with bubbles – this means it's active.

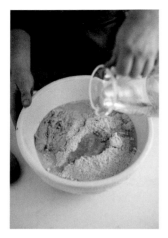

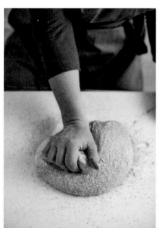

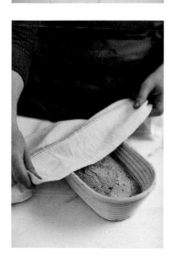

To make the dough

Step 1

Put the dough ingredients into a large bowl and mix thoroughly, then add the active starter mixture and mix.

Step 2

Knead until the dough is smooth and stretchy. Cover and leave for 6–8 hours, folding it a few times throughout this time.

Step 3

Split the dough in half and sit the two halves in the floured proving baskets if using, seam side upwards, or shaped as desired. Cover loosely with a tea towel and leave for 2 hours. Preheat the oven to its highest setting.

Step 4

Turn the loaves out of the baskets onto a baking sheet, so the seam is on the bottom, and transfer the baking sheet directly to the oven. Bake for 5 minutes then turn the oven down to 200°C/400°F/Gas Mark 6 for a further 20–30 minutes. Remove from the oven and transfer to a wire rack to cool.

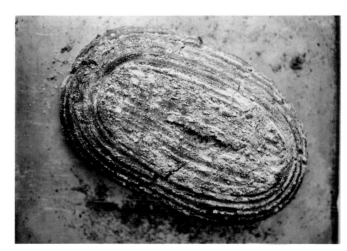

Apple Cider Vinegar
STEP BY STEP

Great for supporting digestion, this type of vinegar is something of a health cure-all. Add a few teaspoons to a glass of water and drink on an empty stomach about 15 minutes before eating, especially before protein-heavy meals. The cider vinegar stimulates our stomach to produce more acid, which is needed to both break down and absorb nutrients from food. Apple cider vinegar has also been clinically proven to reduce the 'bad' form of cholesterol, the sticky sort that can lead to heart disease. Once made, the cider vinegar will keep for up to a year.

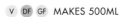 MAKES 500ML

PREP: 15 MINUTES, PLUS FERMENTING TIME (UP TO 6 WEEKS)   11 calories per 15ml

3 organic eating apples
2 tbsp raw honey
About 500ml filtered water at room temperature

Equipment: 2 large sterilised jars, 2 pieces of muslin cloth, 1 elastic band

Step 1

Cut the apples into quarters, reserving the core and pips. Put everything in a sterilised jar – it should come to about halfway up.

Step 2

Add the honey and water and stir well – you can top up with more apple if there's any room.

Step 3

Cover with muslin, secure with the elastic band and leave for 1–2 weeks, then after that stir twice a day using a wooden spoon. It should begin to bubble a little and start to smell of alcohol. This is the beginning of the fermentation process. When this happens, move on to the next step.

Step 4

Strain through a nylon sieve into a large clean jug, then transfer to the second sterilised jar. Cover with a clean piece of muslin and secure with the elastic band. Leave for 3–4 weeks. You will begin to see a film form in the jar. Taste it after about a month. If it needs a little longer, leave it, or if it's too strong add a little filtered water to dilute the taste. When to your liking, strain through a plastic sieve into another clean sterilised jar or bottle.

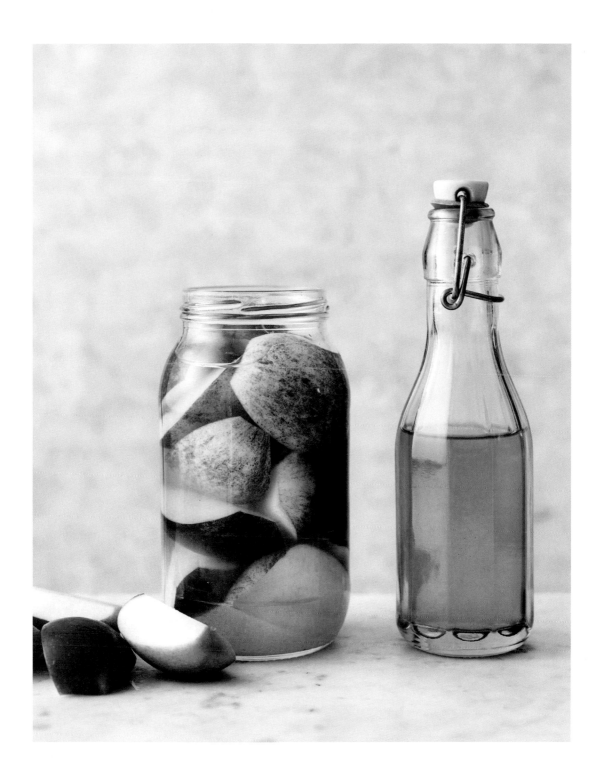

Kombucha
STEP BY STEP

I've been making my own kombucha (fermented green or black tea) brew for well over twenty years. In fact, one of my first television shows was to introduce the delights of kombucha brewing in my cupboard to the unsuspecting actress Lesley Joseph! This is still one of my favourite probiotic drinks to make and I always have a ferment on the go. It's an acquired taste – slightly vinegary, but you'll find it becomes healthily addictive. When I want to curb my alcohol drinking, I simply pour a glass of chilled kombucha into a wineglass and slowly sip with dinner. Perfect.

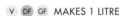 MAKES 1 LITRE

PREP: 15 MINUTES, PLUS FERMENTING TIME (5–18 DAYS)   8 calories per 25ml

3 green or black teabags (it must have a base of 'real' tea)
80g granulated sugar (don't panic – the microbes digest this)
900ml boiling water
Kombucha culture (also called a 'scoby')

Equipment: A 1.5-litre glass jar, 1 muslin cloth

Step 1

Put the teabags in the glass jar, add the sugar and pour in boiling water almost to the top (make sure your glass jar can tolerate boiling water). Stir, leave it for half an hour, then remove the teabags.

Step 2

Now leave it to cool completely, and add your scoby plus any liquid that the scoby comes with. Cover the glass jar with the muslin secured with string and leave it in a spot that's away from direct sunlight and has a steady temperature.

Step 3

Leave the kombucha to ferment; it will take anything between 5 and 18 days. The colour will change slightly and it will become cloudier. Taste, using a small glass – it should taste fruity and tart and maybe a little 'fizzy'. This means it's ready. The longer you leave it, the less sweet it will become and it will begin to taste sour. It depends how you like it.

Step 4

Pour the kombucha through a nylon sieve into a large glass or jug – this is for drinking – leaving behind about a quarter in the jar with the scoby. This is what you will use to make your next brew.

Flavour it ...

To the final juice, add freshly squeezed ginger, raspberries, oranges, lemon or lime, or add to your favourite smoothies or vegetable juice.

What's a scoby?

This stands for Symbiotic Culture Of Bacteria and Yeast.

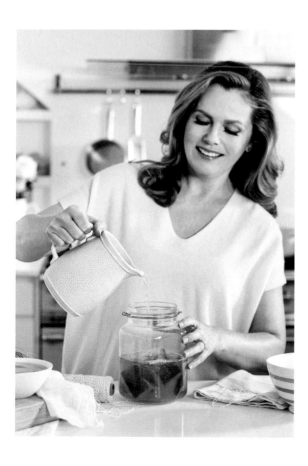

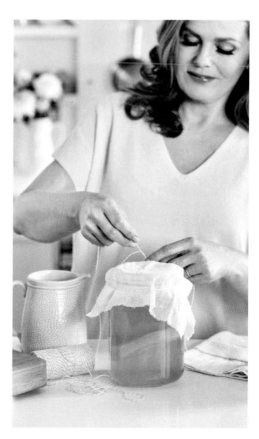

Milk Kefir
STEP BY STEP

Kefir is a staple food in any good-gut regime. It's teeming with beneficial probiotics that can help soothe our gut, and yet for something so powerful, it's so simple to make.

V GF SERVES 1 (2 CUPS); PREP: 10 MINUTES, PLUS FERMENTING TIME (12–48 HOURS); 183 calories

1 tsp milk kefir grains
250ml organic whole (full-fat) milk – look for grass- or pasture-fed

Step 1: Gently rinse the milk kefir grains with fresh milk or spring water and tip them into a sterilised glass jar. Pour in the milk and stir, using a wooden spoon. Loosely cover with the lid, so the gas that is produced can escape while it ferments, or cover with a cloth.

Step 2: Leave it to stand at room temperature for 12–48 hours until it sours to your liking. If you prefer, seal the lid and leave it to ferment in the fridge for a few days, bearing in mind that it will ferment more slowly in a cooler environment.

Step 3: Stir the mixture, then pour it through a plastic sieve into a plastic or glass container. This is then ready to drink, or you can leave it to ripen in a sealed bottle for a little longer, either at room temperature or in the fridge, releasing the lid occasionally to allow the gas to escape.

Step 4: Keep the kefir grains that are in the sieve and start the process again, or you can keep them in a little milk in the fridge for up to a week.

> **LIZ'S TIP**
>
> If you find the taste too sour, you can flavour it with a little raw honey, maple syrup or some blended fruit.

Water Kefir
STEP BY STEP

V GF SERVES 1 (2 CUPS); PREP: 10 MINUTES, PLUS FERMENTING TIME (24–72 HOURS); 160 calories

40g organic unrefined cane sugar, coconut sugar or jaggery (raw sugar)
500ml pure, filtered water
2 tbsp kefir grains

Equipment: 1 large sealable glass jar

Dissolve the sugar in a small amount of hot water in the jar. When it is dissolved add the filtered water, then the kefir grains, and put the lid on. Leave for 24–72 hours, stirring regularly to speed up fermentation. Strain through a plastic sieve, retaining the grains (see Milk Kefir). The kefir water is now ready to drink. Drink as it is or add flavourings such as orange or lemon juice, or use as part of a further recipe.

Dairy Yoghurt
STEP BY STEP

One of the reasons dairy yoghurt hasn't always been so good is because of the added sugar and artificial sweeteners found in so many brands. But when you make it yourself with organic grass-fed milk, you can be assured you're getting a much more nourishing product – and you can flavour it with berries or a little antimicrobial, prebiotic-rich raw honey. Delicious!

 MAKES ABOUT 1 LITRE

PREP: 10 MINUTES, PLUS FERMENTING OVERNIGHT   79 calories (per 100ml)

1 litre whole (full-fat) organic milk
1 tsp powdered milk
50g natural 'live' yoghurt (your starter culture)

Equipment: A cook's thermometer, 1-litre sterilised sealable jar

Step 1

Pour the milk into a pan and heat gently to 45°C – do not boil. If the milk gets too hot it will kill off all the friendly bacteria.

Step 2

Stir in the powdered milk and yoghurt, then spoon it into the jar, seal, cover with a tea towel and put somewhere warm overnight.

Step 3

It should now have thickened into a creamy yoghurt, and the longer you leave it the tangier it will become. Put it in the fridge and leave it to chill before eating. It will keep for up to 1 week in the fridge.

LIZ'S TIP

I like to add the contents of a good probiotic capsule to my starter culture to enrich the yoghurt. Remember to always retain a little of your yoghurt to make the next batch and keep the microbes going.

Sauerkraut
STEP BY STEP

Simply fermented veggies, sauerkraut is a bit like a tart coleslaw and is such a great way to get raw vegetables into our diet. Not only is the fibre good for bowel health but the fermentation means that all those good bugs will help support the growth of even more. All you need is one tablespoon a day as a topping or side dish. It adds a sharpness to salads and goes really well with a hot buttered potato – yummy!

 MAKES ABOUT 1KG

PREP: 20 MINUTES, PLUS FERMENTING TIME (3–16 DAYS)   11 calories (per 25g)

1 white cabbage, about 2kg, finely shredded   *Equipment:* A 1-litre sterilised sealable jar
1 tbsp sea salt

Step 1

Put the cabbage into a large glass or ceramic bowl, add the salt and massage it all together with your hands, coating well.

Step 2

Now pound the cabbage – a good thing to use for this is the pestle from a pestle and mortar or the round end of a rolling pin. Squash and pound it for about 5–10 minutes until plenty of water is released.

Step 3

Spoon the cabbage, a little at a time, into the sterilised jar, squashing it down as you go, using the pestle or rolling pin, and making sure it's tightly packed.

Step 4

Make sure the cabbage is fully immersed under the water – it needs this to ferment properly. Secure the lid and leave for 3–16 days in the kitchen, or longer if you like a stronger flavour. The process will be slower if you prefer it to ferment in your fridge.

Red Cabbage and Fennel Seed Sauerkraut

33 calories (per 25g)

2kg red cabbage, finely shredded
1 tbsp sea salt
1 tsp fennel seeds or caraway seeds

Make this in the same way as you would the white cabbage sauerkraut.

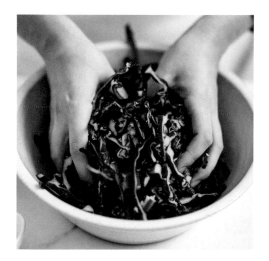
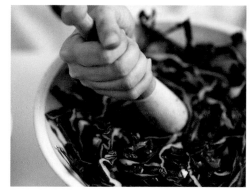
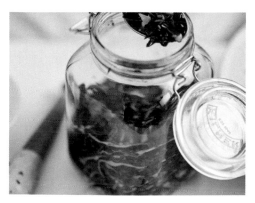
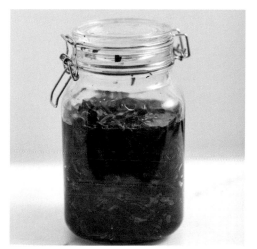

Kimchi
STEP BY STEP

Once made, you can keep this fermented superstar for up to 12 months. Place it in the fridge to stop the fermentation process; the taste will be tangier and the spices will mellow over time. The trick to tell whether or not your kimchi is ready to eat is in the taste – when it isn't yet ready and fully ripe, you'll be able to taste and smell the individual ingredients as they haven't had time to do their thing. As they mingle and start to ferment, the flavours begin to blend together and the kimchi will taste sour with a slight zing to it. It will also have the pungent smell that is unique to kimchi.

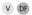 MAKES ABOUT 2KG

PREP: 20 MINUTES, PLUS OVERNIGHT DRYING,

AND FERMENTING TIME (ABOUT 3–7 DAYS)   5 calories (per 25g)

4 litres spring water

4 tbsp sea salt

2 Chinese cabbages (also known as 'nappa cabbages'), about 1kg each

1 bunch spring onions, trimmed and finely sliced

10cm piece fresh ginger, peeled and finely grated

5 large cloves garlic, peeled and grated or finely chopped

½ eating apple, peeled and finely sliced

2 tbsp dried chilli flakes

2 tbsp hot pepper paste (available at Asian stores)

Equipment: 1 large bowl, 2 × 1-litre sterilised sealable jars

Step 1

First make the brine: put the water and salt into a large bowl, or use two. Stir so that the salt disperses into the water. Trim the bases of the cabbages, then slice lengthways into quarters and add to the bowl, making sure all the cabbage is immersed in the water. Leave for 1–2 hours so the salt can penetrate it.

Step 2

Drain the cabbage really well, pat dry, then leave it to dry overnight.

Step 3

In a large bowl put the spring onions, ginger, garlic, apple, chilli flakes and hot pepper paste and mix well until combined. Now add the cabbage a little at a time, stirring as you go – you can chop it a little if you wish, but leave it fairly chunky as it's best chopped as you use it. Turn the mixture really well in the bowl (using food-preparation gloves helps here) until everything is completely coated.

Step 4

Add the mixture to the sterilised jars, pressing it down as you go so it's well packed. The cabbage needs to be submerged under the juice. Don't pack to the top of the jars because as it ferments and expands it may try to overflow. Seal with the lid and leave for up to 3 days in warm weather and up to 7 days in cold, before using.

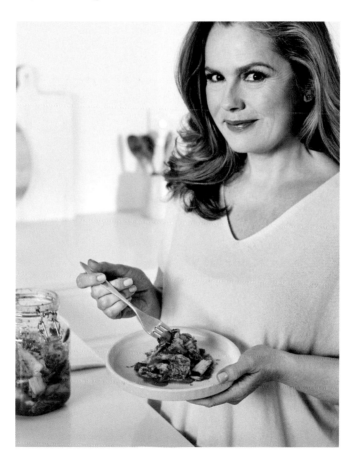

BREAKFAST AND BRUNCH

Vanilla Overnight Oats

The beauty of soaking oats, nuts and seeds overnight is that it starts off the germination process and softens all the ingredients – that means there's virtually zero prep needed in the morning and everything is also easier to digest.

 SERVES 4

PREP: OVERNIGHT SOAKING AND CHILLING   303 calories

150g organic porridge oats

200g plain live yoghurt

1 capful real vanilla extract (or the scrapings of a vanilla pod)

200ml Milk Kefir (page 106) or organic milk

2 tsp pumpkin seeds

10 almonds, with skin on, halved lengthways (or use blanched almonds if these are easier to tolerate)

1 organic eating apple per serving, cored and sliced for topping

- Tip the oats into a large bowl or sealable container. Mix the yoghurt with the vanilla extract and add along with the kefir or milk. Stir well to combine.

- Add the pumpkin seeds and almonds and stir well. Cover the bowl or seal the lid and put in the fridge overnight.

- Serve the next day, topped with the sliced apple.

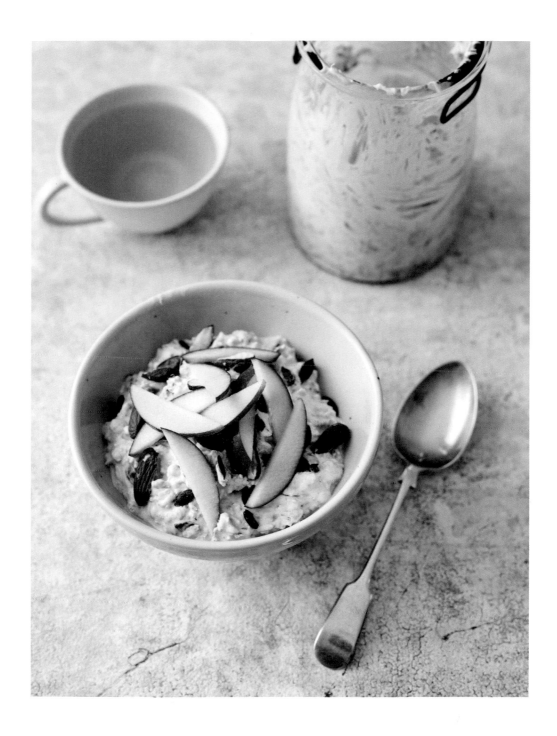

Raspberry Buckwheat Porridge

This pseudo-grain (it's actually a type of grass seed) is rich in the mineral magnesium, which helps our blood vessels relax, making buckwheat ideal as part of a calming, de-stressing diet. The berries add an anthocyanin antioxidant boost and pumpkin seeds help combat bad bugs. Goji berries are especially gut-friendly as they help feed our good bugs.

  V DF GF SERVES 1   392 calories

80g buckwheat
220ml almond milk (or milk of choice)

For the topping:
1 tsp pumpkin seeds
1 tsp dried goji berries
8 raspberries

- Put the buckwheat and almond milk into a small pan, and cook on a low heat, stirring occasionally. Cook for about 15–20 minutes until it begins to thicken. If it needs it, add a little hot water to loosen.

- When the buckwheat is tender and cooked, spoon out into a bowl and top with the pumpkin seeds, goji berries and raspberries.

> **LIZ'S TIP**
>
> Add a teaspoon of raw or manuka honey if you like this a little sweeter.

Coconut and Banana Porridge

Both oats and bananas contain prebiotic fibres to support our digestion – and it's just such a delicious combination.

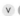 V DF SERVES 2   244 calories

100g organic porridge oats
200ml coconut milk (check no added sugar)
200ml filtered water
1 small banana, sliced

- Tip the porridge oats into a pan and add the coconut milk and water, bring to a slow boil, then reduce to a simmer, stirring continually.

- Cook for about 4–5 minutes or until the porridge is creamy. If it starts to thicken too much, top up with a little hot water.

- Spoon into a bowl and top with the sliced banana.

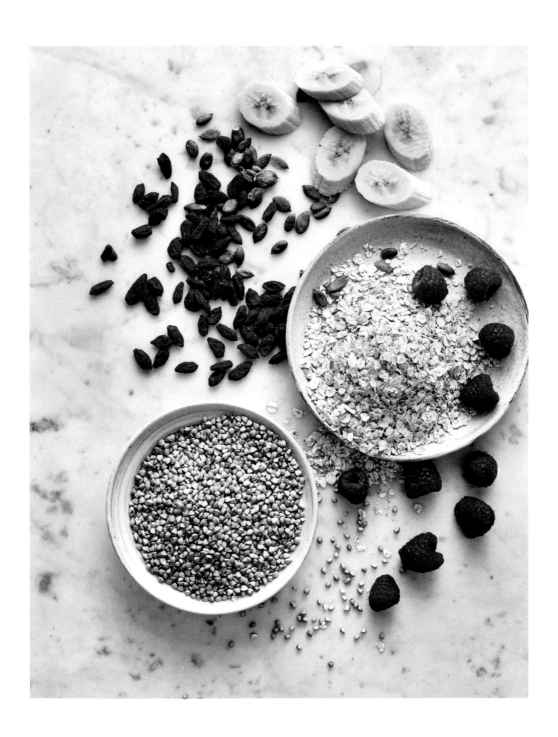

Oat and Berry Breakfast Bar

These delicious breakfast bars are jam-packed with pro- and prebiotics, and the addition of chia seeds supplies healthy Omega-3 fats. It makes a delicious snack at any time.

ⓥ MAKES 14 SLICES

PREP: OVERNIGHT CHILLING   115 calories

90g pack coconut chunks
200g organic porridge oats
40g chia seeds
1 tbsp almond butter
2 tbsp raw honey (unprocessed, not heat-treated)
1 tbsp plain Greek yoghurt
150g blueberries

For the topping:
1 tbsp plain Greek yoghurt
1 capful real vanilla extract (or the scrapings of a vanilla pod)

- Preheat the oven to 200°C/400°F/Gas Mark 6. Put the coconut chunks in a small (about 29 × 19cm) lightly greased baking tin, then put in the oven for 10–15 minutes or until golden. Remove and leave to cool a little, then finely chop and set aside.

- Meanwhile, into a large bowl put the oats and chia seeds, the almond butter and honey, and beat together until the oats are well combined. Add the yoghurt and mix again, then tip in the blueberries and cooled coconut and stir well.

- Line the tin with parchment paper, leaving the edges overlapping, then spoon in the oat mixture, spread over the tin until even and pack it down well using the back of a wooden spoon. Put in the oven and bake for 20–25 minutes or until golden brown. Remove from the oven and leave to cool completely.

- For the topping, mix the yoghurt and vanilla extract together, then spoon it over the oat and blueberry slab in a drizzle effect. Put in the fridge overnight or for a few hours to chill and set, then slice, to serve.

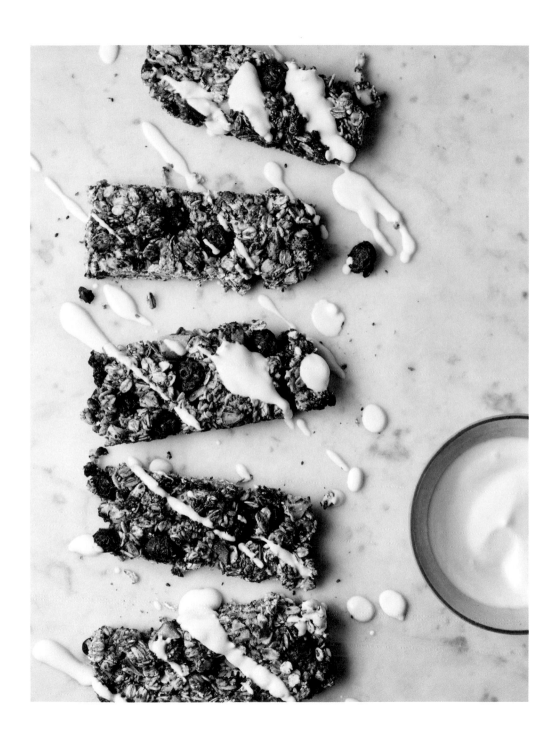

Buttermilk Pancakes Topped with Cherries and Yoghurt

Buttermilk is slightly fermented, so it's easier to digest; raw honey in this recipe adds a prebiotic boost, while the coconut oil is rich in fats that help protect the lining of your gut. A perfect weekend brunch for all the family.

v MAKES 6–8   222–167 calories

160g self-raising flour   For the topping:
1 tsp bicarbonate of soda   150g fresh or frozen cherries, stoned
285ml buttermilk   About 3 tbsp natural live Greek yoghurt
1 organic egg
1 tbsp raw honey (unprocessed, non heat-treated)
About 50g organic butter or solid coconut oil

- Into a large bowl put the flour and bicarbonate of soda and mix well. In a jug mix together the buttermilk, egg and honey until well combined.

- Pour the buttermilk mixture into the flour and beat together using a wooden spoon. Be careful not to over-beat – it can have a few lumps in it. Chill the mixture in the fridge for 20 minutes.

- Heat a little of the butter or coconut oil at a time in a small non-stick frying or crêpe pan, using just enough to coat the base of the pan. When the butter or coconut oil is hot, add a generous tablespoon of the mixture and spread it out a little. Turn the heat down to low and leave it to cook for about 3–4 minutes or until the underside starts to turn golden and it's firm enough to flip over using a wide spatula or fish slice. Cook the other side for about the same time or until the mixture is cooked through. Remove from the pan and keep warm while you cook the rest of the pancakes (30 minutes altogether).

- Heat the cherries in a pan, squashing them slightly with a wooden spoon. When heated through, spoon a little on top of each pancake along with a dollop of the Greek yoghurt.

LIZ'S TIP

If you can't tolerate wheat very well, make this using a gluten-free flour or try spelt flour.

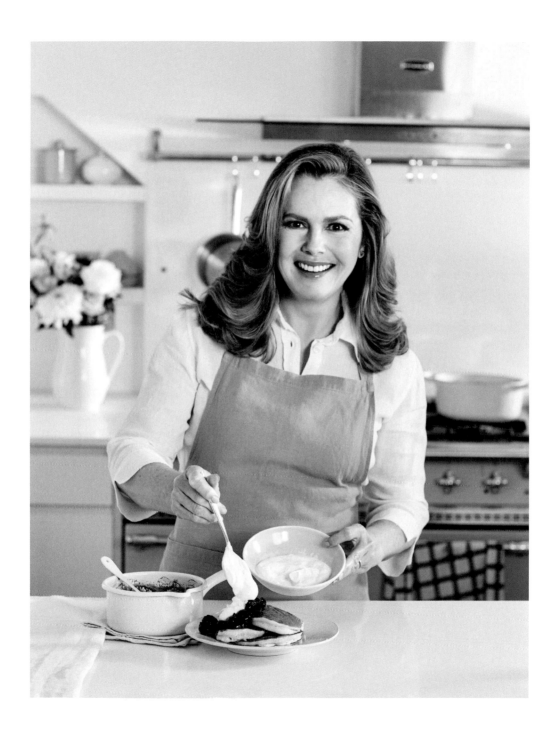

Roasted Tempeh with Turmeric Eggs, Kale and Avocado

Unlike a lot of processed soy products, traditionally made tempeh is fermented, meaning your gut shouldn't have problems digesting it. The kale ramps up the prebiotic content and the super-spice turmeric makes this a powerful anti-inflammatory dish, perfect for a hearty weekend brunch.

v SERVES 4   500 calories

200g kale, tough stalks removed
400g tempeh, sliced into lengths
1 tbsp extra virgin olive or rapeseed oil
Splash tamari soy sauce
4 organic eggs

Sea salt and freshly ground black pepper
25g organic butter
1–2 tsp turmeric
2 ripe avocados, halved, stoned and sliced

- Preheat the oven to 200°C/400°F/Gas Mark 6. Put the kale into a steamer or a metal colander over a pan of simmering water, put the lid on and steam for about 15–20 minutes or until just tender. Remove and set aside.

- Toss the tempeh with the olive oil and tamari sauce and put in a roasting tin, then into the oven, and cook for about 10–15 minutes or until it's beginning to turn crisp and golden. Remove and set aside.

- Lightly beat the eggs together and season well. Heat the butter, and when melted add the egg mix and move it around the pan with a fork. Stir in the turmeric and cook for a few seconds more – it should still look creamy and slightly undercooked.

- Remove it from the heat and divide between serving plates. Add the tempeh and kale and top with the avocado slices, to serve.

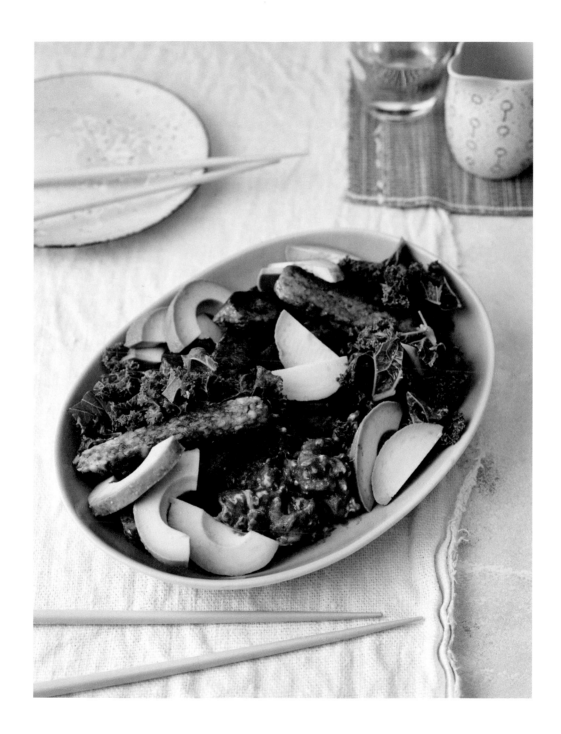

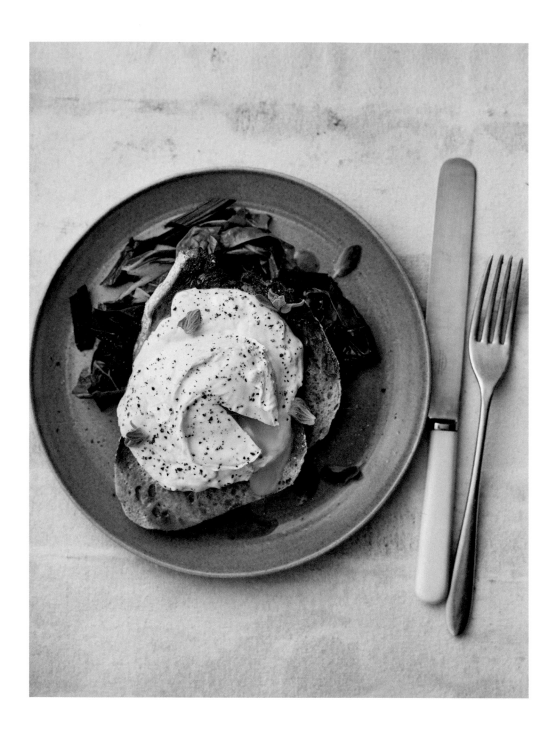

Turkish Eggs with Yoghurt and Tahini

This sumptuous breakfast may just be my new 'avocado on toast'. It's a gut-healing take on eggs Benedict, but with an antimicrobial twist courtesy of the garlic and turmeric. What's more, it's super-simple to prepare – enjoy!

v   SERVES 2   303 calories

1 heaped tbsp plain Greek yoghurt
Sea salt and freshly ground black pepper
1–2 cloves garlic, grated
1–2 tsp tahini
25g organic butter
1 tsp turmeric

2 organic eggs
2 slices spelt or rye sourdough, toasted
Handful of fresh oregano leaves, to garnish
   (optional)
About 8 leaves of rainbow chard, steamed, to
   serve

- Add the yoghurt to a bowl, season well with the sea salt and freshly ground black pepper and stir in the grated garlic and tahini. Taste, and adjust the seasoning as needed. Set aside.

- Bring a small pan of salted water to the boil ready for the eggs. Meanwhile, melt the butter in a small pan and stir in the turmeric until smooth. Put to one side and keep warm. Crack the eggs into the water and cook until poached.

- Drizzle the melted turmeric butter over the sourdough, then spoon on the yoghurt and top with the poached eggs and a few oregano leaves (if using). Serve with the steamed chard.

Tray Bake All-in-One Breakfast

Who can resist the simplicity of a tray bake? Cut up all the ingredients, throw them into a pan, drizzle over the oil and pop it in the oven – et voilà! A gut-healing meal in minutes thanks to prebiotic asparagus, parasite-fighting oregano, healthy-fat-filled olive oil and a slice of sourdough. The smoked salmon is an optional indulgence.

 SERVES 4   187 calories

150g asparagus spears, trimmed
250g button mushrooms
300g cherry tomatoes
Sea salt and freshly ground black pepper

A few stalks fresh oregano, leaves only
1 tbsp extra virgin olive or rapeseed oil
250g wild smoked salmon (optional)
Toasted spelt or rye sourdough bread, to serve

- Preheat the oven to 200°C/400°F/Gas Mark 6.

- Put the asparagus, mushrooms and tomatoes into a roasting tin. Season well with the sea salt and freshly ground black pepper, then scatter over the oregano leaves, drizzle with the oil and toss everything together with your hands.

- Put in the oven and cook for about 20 minutes or until the vegetables are beginning to char slightly and the tomatoes are starting to burst.

- Remove from the oven and transfer to serving plates. Serve with smoked salmon (if using) and toasted sourdough bread.

LIZ'S TIP

Look for wild smoked salmon whenever possible, as farmed salmon (even organic) comes from caged salmon treated with sea-louse medication.

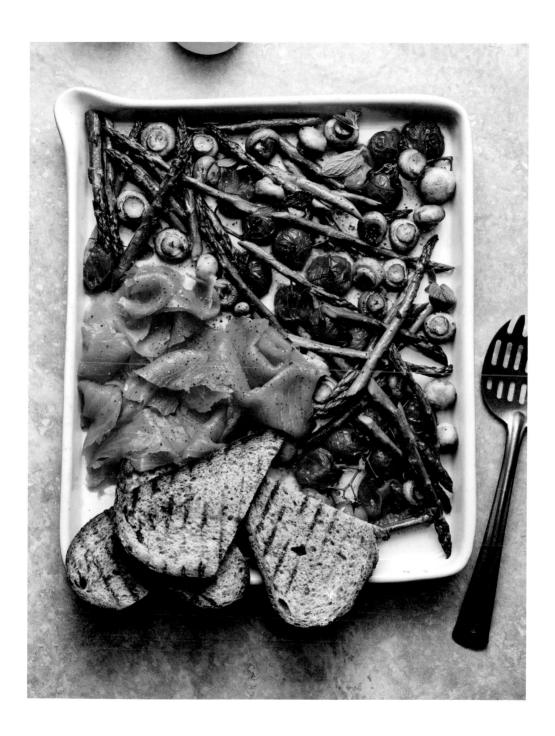

Sweet Potato Rösti with Poached Eggs

If breakfast isn't really breakfast without hash browns, then this one's for you. The addition of chicory and onion to this sweet potato rösti ramps up the prebiotic fibre content, while the oozing poached eggs and tart, crunchy kimchi balance each other perfectly.

 MAKES 8   182 calories

600g sweet potatoes, peeled and roughly grated
200g chicory, trimmed and finely shredded
Sea salt and freshly ground black pepper
3 tbsp extra virgin olive or rapeseed oil
1 onion, finely chopped

2 cloves garlic, finely chopped
5–6 organic eggs
About 2 tbsp Kimchi (page 110; optional)

- Put the sweet potatoes and chicory into a large bowl and season well with the sea salt and freshly ground black pepper.

- Heat 1 tbsp of the oil in a frying pan and add the onion. Cook for 2–3 minutes until softened, then stir in the garlic and cook for a minute more. Tip this into the sweet potato mixture and leave it to cool, then add one of the eggs and mix well. If you think the mixture needs another egg, add it and stir again. You may want to season it again too.

- Heat a little of the remaining oil in a large non-stick frying pan. Scoop out a handful of the mixture and pat it together with your hands to form a cake. Carefully add to the pan – two at a time are probably enough to do at once. Cook undisturbed on a low heat for about 5–8 minutes, or until they are beginning to firm up and the undersides are starting to turn golden. Flip over and cook for a further 5 minutes or until golden and cooked through. Remove from the pan and keep warm while you cook the remaining mixture.

- While they are cooking, add the remaining eggs one at a time to a pan of simmering water until poached. Remove with a slotted spoon. Transfer the röstis to serving plates, top with a poached egg and serve with a little kimchi on the side (if using).

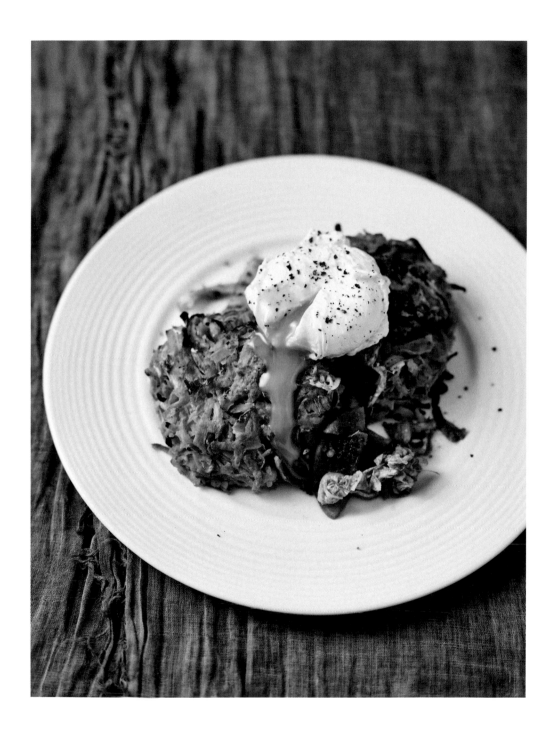

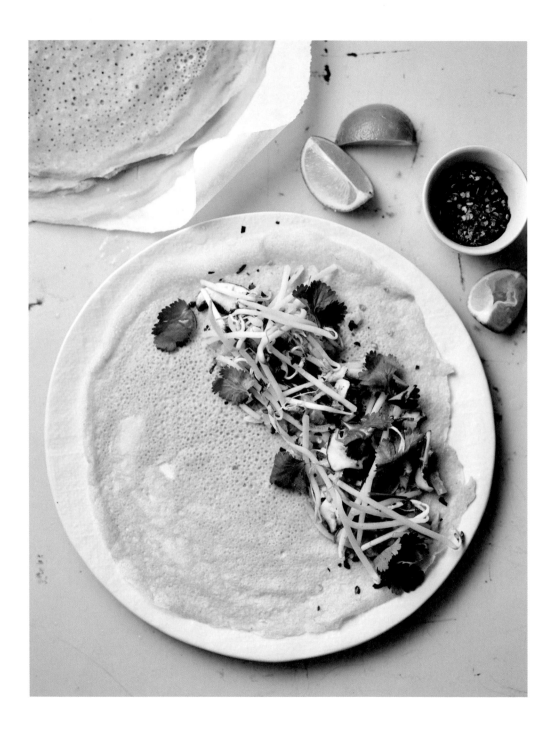

Vietnamese Turmeric Pancakes

Just because I love pancakes, here's another take on them but this time made from rice flour, which is gluten-free, with my favourite super-spice turmeric thrown in for added colour and flavour.

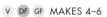 MAKES 4–6   190–126 calories

For the pancakes:
100g rice flour
1 egg
1 tsp turmeric
Pinch sea salt
100ml coconut milk
200ml water
Drizzle of olive or rapeseed oil

For the filling:
Drizzle of sesame oil
1 Chinese (nappa) cabbage, or use a pointed
    green cabbage, shredded
Sea salt and freshly ground black pepper
150g chestnut mushrooms, finely sliced
5cm piece fresh ginger, peeled and grated
Pinch chilli flakes (optional)
2 tsp rice vinegar
1 lime
Handful of coriander (optional)
Handful of beansprouts

- First make the pancakes by putting the rice flour, egg, turmeric and pinch of sea salt into a bowl. Pour in the coconut milk and water and whisk until smooth. Place in the fridge to rest.

- Now make the filling. Heat the sesame oil in a wok, add the cabbage, season and stir-fry, then add the mushrooms, ginger and chilli flakes (if using), and toss everything around the wok. Cook for a couple of minutes until the cabbage is starting to wilt, then add the rice vinegar and cook for a few minutes more. Taste, adjust the seasoning if necessary, remove from the heat and put to one side. You can reheat it again when the pancakes are ready, if necessary.

- To prepare the pancakes, brush the bottom of a flat non-stick frying pan or a crêpe pan with the olive oil and heat gently, then add a ladleful of the batter and swirl it around the pan to coat. Leave to cook undisturbed for a minute, then loosen around the edges, and continue to cook for about 3 more minutes or until the pancake starts to crisp up around the edges.

- Transfer it to a serving plate, pile some cabbage mixture onto one half of the pancake and garnish with a squeeze of lime, coriander (if using) and beansprouts. Fold the pancake over, to serve. Repeat until all the batter is used – it depends on how thin you want your pancakes as to how many the mixture will make.

SNACKS

Beetroot and Roquefort Muffins

These savoury muffins are packed with protein so will help keep you fuller for longer. I love making a batch at the weekend, then having them to hand during a busy week. A great way to keep hunger pangs at bay.

MAKES 10   243 calories

300g organic wholegrain spelt flour
2 tsp baking powder
½ tsp bicarbonate of soda
1 tsp chopped fresh oregano
Sea salt and freshly ground black pepper
100ml olive or rapeseed oil
100ml plain live yoghurt

100ml organic whole (full-fat) milk
2 organic eggs
100g Roquefort cheese, crumbled
3 small cooked beetroots, grated

Equipment: A large 12-hole muffin tin lined with
    10 large paper cases

- Preheat the oven to 190°C/375°F/Gas Mark 5.

- Put the flour, baking powder, bicarbonate of soda, oregano and a pinch of sea salt and freshly ground black pepper into a bowl and stir.

- Into another bowl put the oil, yoghurt, milk, eggs and cheese and mix well. Tip the mixture into the flour and stir briefly, then add the beetroot and stir until combined. Do not beat until smooth – it's OK for it to be a little lumpy.

- Divide the mixture between the muffin cases in the tin, and put in the oven for 25–30 minutes until risen and golden. Remove from the oven and transfer the muffins to a wire rack to cool.

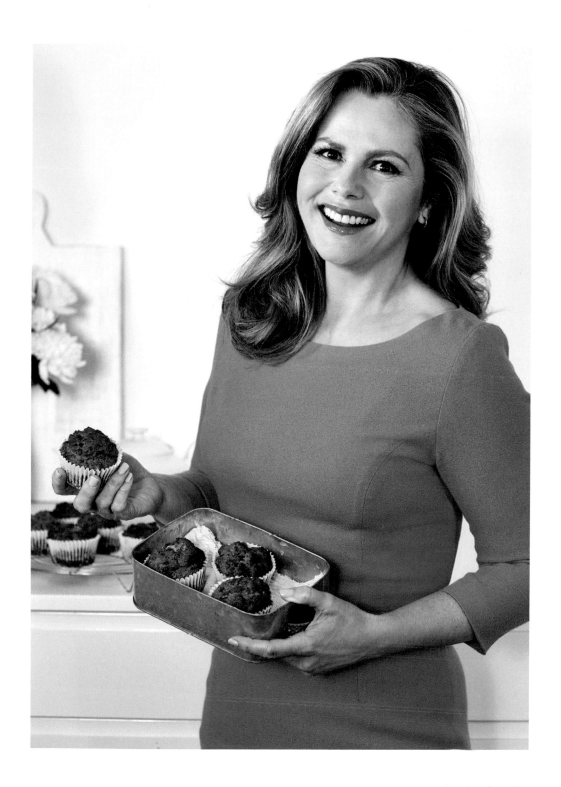

Spiced Apple Crisps

For a sweet treat with added crunch, these apple and ginger crisps hit the spot nicely. Spiced with cinnamon to boost our metabolism and keep bad bacteria at bay, they're a tasty snack that's so simple to make.

V DF GF SERVES 4–6   80–54 calories

6 firm eating apples (leave the peel on), preferably
   organic, individually sliced very finely (use a
   mandolin if you have one)
Fine sprinkle of ground ginger or cinnamon

- Preheat the oven to 160°C/325°F/Gas Mark 3.

- Sit the apples on a baking sheet lined with parchment paper, leaving space between. Lightly dust with the ground ginger or cinnamon and put in the oven.

- Bake for 45 minutes, but keep an eye on them to make sure they don't over-colour. They should be pale golden and will start to curl up around the edges. Remove from the oven and leave to cool on the baking sheet for 5 minutes, then carefully slide them away with a palette knife. When cool, store in a sealed container for up to 3 days.

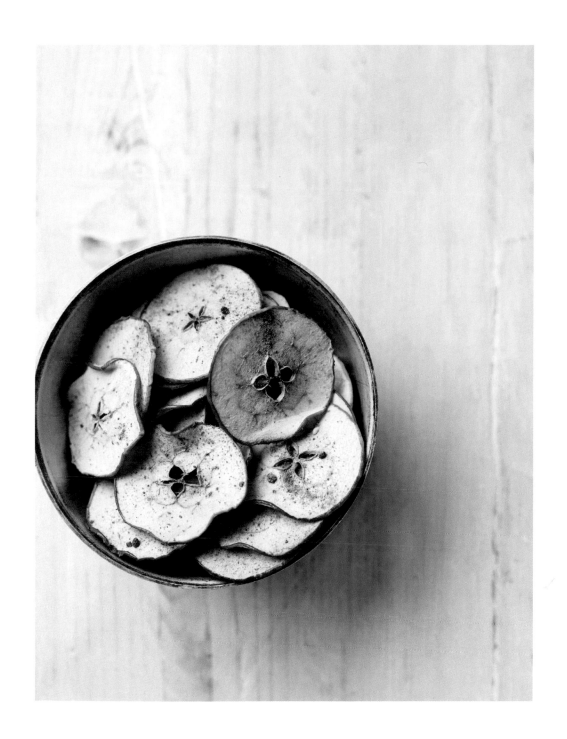

Fermented Tea and Pumpkin Seed Crackers with Asparagus Pâté

The asparagus pâté provides a prebiotic treat for your good bugs. Try soaking the pumpkin seeds overnight to make them more digestible, before adding them to this fermented tea cracker recipe. I've served here with the Fennel Slaw from page 140.

ᵥ MAKES ABOUT 30
PREP: OVERNIGHT SOAKING
64 calories

120g organic wholegrain spelt flour
1 tsp dried oregano
1 tbsp pumpkin seeds
50g ground flax seeds (linseed)
1½ tsp black sesame seeds
Sea salt and freshly ground black pepper
80g organic butter, cubed
100ml Kombucha (fermented black or green tea; page 104), or use Apple Cider Vinegar (page102)

For the asparagus pâté:
200g asparagus tips, trimmed
2 tbsp plain Greek yoghurt
A few fresh oregano leaves
Sea salt and freshly ground black pepper

- First make the asparagus pâté. Steam the asparagus tips in a steamer or sit them in a metal colander, covered, over a pan of simmering water. Cook for about 4–5 minutes or until tender. Remove, leave to cool, then roughly chop and put them in a food processor. Add the yoghurt, oregano, sea salt and freshly ground black pepper, then whizz until blended. Taste, and season some more if required. Keep covered in the fridge until ready to use.

- Now make the crackers. Preheat the oven to 170°C/350°F/Gas Mark 4. Put into a bowl the flour, oregano, pumpkin seeds, flax seeds, black sesame seeds and sea salt and freshly ground black pepper. Mix well to combine.

- Add the butter and rub the mixture with your fingertips until it resembles breadcrumbs and starts to come together as a dough. Now add the kombucha and mix – it will be quite wet, so use your hands to squish it all together.

- Turn the wet dough out onto a baking sheet lined with parchment paper and use a palette knife to spread it out smoothly to cover the sheet, then score it into about 30 squares (each one 6 × 6cm). Put in the oven and bake for about 20–25 minutes or until crispy and golden. Remove from the oven and leave to cool completely, before removing from the paper with the palette knife. Serve with the asparagus pâté. The crackers will keep in a sealed container for up to 1 week.

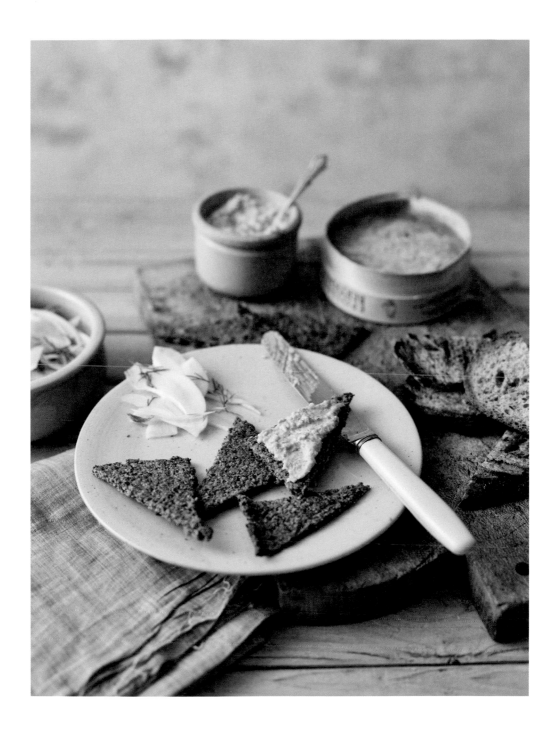

Rye Sourdough with Époisses and Fennel Slaw

Mmmmm, runny cheese! Époisses is a favourite of mine: stinky, sticky and very spreadable. Add it to fibre-rich sourdough and prebiotic-packed slaw for a winning combination.

SERVES 4   286 calories

2 tsp extra virgin olive or rapeseed oil
4 slices organic wholemeal rye sourdough
200g Époisses cheese (at room temperature)

For the fennel slaw:
1 small fennel bulb, trimmed and finely sliced
2 tsp apple cider vinegar
Sea salt and freshly ground black pepper
1 tsp fresh dill, chopped

- First make the fennel slaw. Put the fennel into a bowl, drizzle with the apple cider vinegar and season well with the sea salt and freshly ground black pepper. Stir in the dill and put the mixture aside for the flavours to mingle.

- Heat a griddle pan to hot, drizzle the olive oil over the sourdough, then put a couple of slices at a time into the pan and toast for a few minutes until char lines appear, then turn and do the other side. Repeat with the remaining slices.

- Spread the Époisses over the toasted bread and serve with the fennel slaw on the side.

Sourdough Bruschetta with Seasonal Toppings

There are plenty of things you can do with sourdough, including topping it with a variety of seasonal veggies. Eating with the seasons often means enjoying fresher, more locally grown produce. Vegetables eaten in season tend to have fewer post-harvest chemical residues, as they have not been kept in storage. Unpasteurised cheese is not recommended if you are pregnant or have a compromised immune system.

V SERVES 2

2 slices Spelt Sourdough (page 100)
Drizzle of extra virgin olive oil

1 clove garlic

- Brush the sourdough all over with the olive oil, then rub the garlic over the slices. Heat a griddle pan to hot and add the sourdough. Toast until the underside starts to turn golden and char lines appear, then turn and cook the other side until golden. Remove, and spoon on the topping.

Spring Topping: Asparagus and Goat's Cheese

V SERVES 2   461 calories

200g asparagus tips, trimmed
Sea salt and freshly ground black pepper
Drizzle of extra virgin olive oil

100g unpasteurised soft goat's cheese
A few thyme leaves, to garnish

- Season the asparagus with the sea salt and freshly ground black pepper, then toss with the olive oil. Heat a griddle pan to hot, then add the asparagus and cook for 3–4 minutes or until the underside begins to char, then turn and cook the other side until golden and char lines appear. Remove, and top the toasted sourdough, then crumble over the cheese and sprinkle with the thyme leaves, to serve.

Summer Topping: Courgette, Garlic and Shaved Fennel

v SERVES 2   351 calories

2 small courgettes, sliced with a T-peeler
Sea salt and freshly ground black pepper
1 clove garlic, grated
A few oregano leaves

Zest and juice of ½ small lemon
½ small fennel, trimmed and very finely shaved
1 tsp Apple Cider Vinegar (page 102)
Drizzle of olive oil (optional)

- Season the courgettes with sea salt and freshly ground black pepper, then toss with the garlic, oregano and lemon zest and juice. Toss the fennel with the apple cider vinegar and season well.

- Heat a griddle pan to hot, add the courgette strips a few at a time so as not to overcrowd the pan. Cook for a minute or so until char lines appear on the underside, then turn and cook the other side. Repeat until all the courgette is cooked.

- Pile the courgettes onto the sourdough toast – then, to serve, top the lot with the shaved fennel. You can lightly char the fennel also, if you wish, in which case toss with the olive oil first. But it is nice served fresh over the griddled courgettes.

Autumn Topping: Mushrooms and Sage with Apple Cider Vinegar

v SERVES 2   295 calories

Drizzle of extra virgin olive oil
40g chestnut mushrooms, finely sliced
Sea salt and freshly ground black pepper
1 clove garlic, finely chopped

2 sage leaves, roughly chopped
1 tsp apple cider vinegar (page 102)
1 tsp finely chopped flat-leaf parsley

- Heat the olive oil in a small frying pan, add the mushrooms, season well with the sea salt and freshly ground black pepper, and cook for a few minutes until they start to release their juices. Then throw in the garlic and sage and stir. Cook for a further minute, stirring so the garlic and sage don't burn. Add the apple cider vinegar, turn the heat up a little and toss, then remove from the heat, add the parsley and turn to coat.

- Spoon the mixture onto the toasted sourdough and serve.

Winter Topping: Kale with Poached Pear and Gorgonzola

SERVES 2   430 calories

Handful of kale leaves, tough stalks removed   Sea salt and freshly ground black pepper
Juice of ¼ lemon   1 dessert pear, peeled
Pinch chilli flakes (optional)   About 50g Gorgonzola, crumbled

- Steam the kale for about 15–20 minutes or until tender, then toss with the lemon juice and chilli flakes (if using) and season with the sea salt and freshly ground black pepper.

- While the kale is cooking put the pear in a pan of water and simmer gently until tender, then remove and slice. Spoon the kale onto the toasted sourdough and top with the warm pear slices and Gorgonzola.

LIZ'S TIP

I find that making small amounts of simple snacks and canapés are a good way to introduce new foods or flavours to the family. Children especially like the idea of small, crunchy bites and these unusual combos are easier to start slipping into the family's dietary list of 'likes' when introduced little and often. Grown-up fussy eaters are also more likely to come around to loving these gut-food heroes when they are presented as a treat alongside a glass of something special.

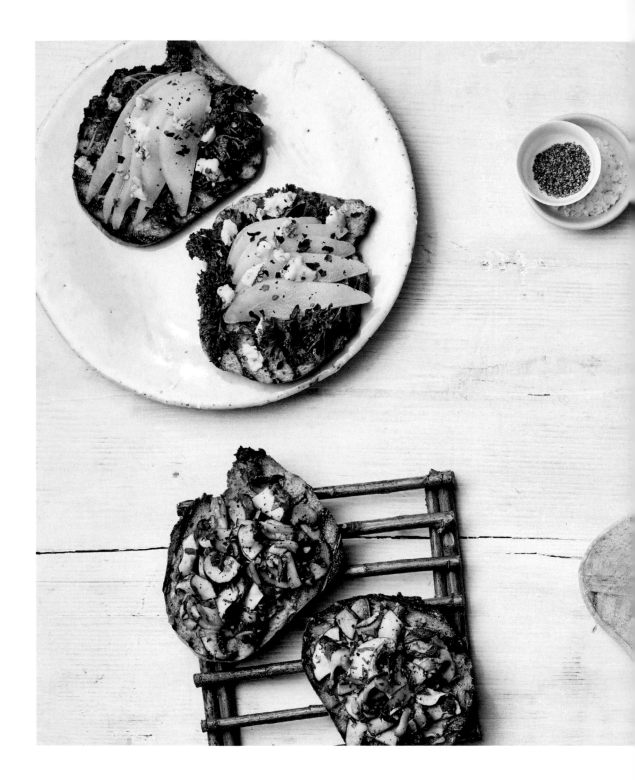

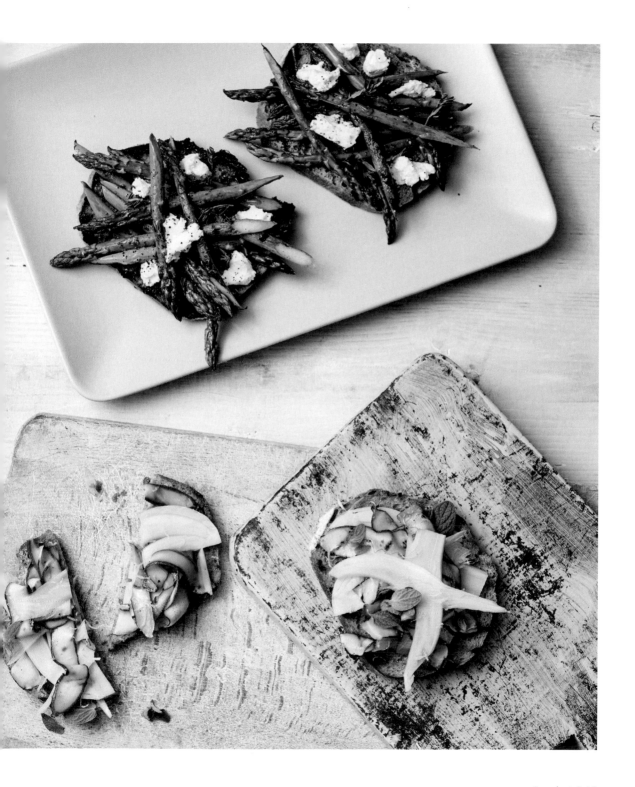

Beetroot Dip with Fermented Carrots

Children of all ages love raw carrot sticks, and here's a new way to enjoy them. Fermented veg take a little time to prepare, but are well worth it as you'll have tummy-friendly snacks that are easier on the digestion. Make a big batch – the carrots will keep for around 6 weeks. Plus, beetroot for the dip is a great energy booster.

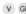 BEETROOT DIP: SERVES 4–6
CARROTS: MAKES A 1-LITRE JAR
PREP: 20 MINUTES, PLUS FERMENTING TIME (7–8 DAYS)   80–54 calories

For the fermented carrots:
About 1.6 litres filtered water
3 tbsp sea salt
800g organic carrots, peeled and quartered
    lengthways, any chunky ones sliced again into
    finer strips
Sprig of dill
100ml Water Kefir (page 106)

For the beetroot dip:
1kg fresh beetroots, stalks trimmed
1 tsp caraway seeds
1 tbsp extra virgin olive or rapeseed oil
2 cloves garlic, grated
Juice of ¼–½ lime
Sea salt and freshly ground black pepper

- To ferment the carrots, add half the water to a large non-metallic bowl, then add 1 tbsp of the salt. Stir with a wooden spoon, then add the carrots and more water to cover. Set aside and leave overnight.

- Drain the carrots well, then pack them into a 1-litre sterilised sealable jar and add the dill. In a glass or plastic jug mix together the water kefir, the rest of the salt and about 400ml of the filtered water. Give it a stir with a wooden spoon and pour over the carrots.

- Seal the lid and leave for at least 1 week before using. Eat the fermented carrots as a healthy snack on their own or serve with the beetroot dip.

- To make the beetroot dip, preheat the oven to 200°C/400°F/Gas Mark 6. Put the beetroots in a roasting tin, cover with cold water, then cover the tin with foil. Put in the oven and cook for 1 hour or until the beetroots are tender when poked with a knife. Remove from the oven, drain and leave to cool, then peel away the skins. Put to one side.

• Put the caraway seeds into a food processor and blitz, then add the cooled beetroots, the olive oil, garlic and lime juice, and season well with the sea salt and freshly ground black pepper. Whizz until puréed, taste, and adjust the seasoning as needed. Transfer to a bowl and serve at room temperature. It will keep, covered, in the fridge for up to 4 days.

LIZ'S TIP

You can ferment any vegetables you like, according to what is in season.

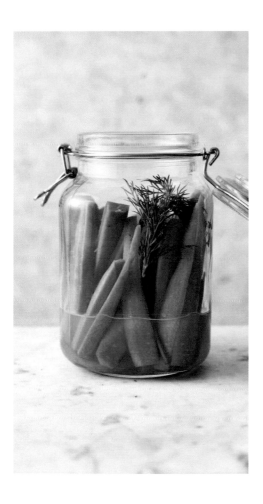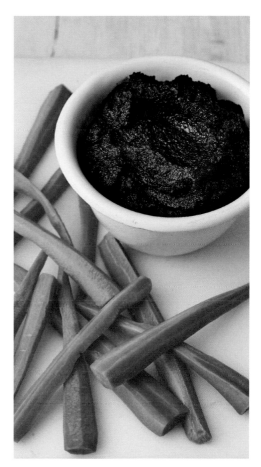

Seaweed and Miso Bites

Algae truly deserve their status as a vitamin- and mineral-packed superfood. They are reputed to assist with the removal of toxins from the body, and those used for cooking – here I'm using nori – provide valuable amounts of iodine, so it's a great addition to these gut-friendly, tasty bites.

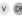 V DF **MAKES ABOUT 34 BITES**   36 calories

200g organic wholemeal rye flour
Freshly ground black pepper
2 tsp chia seeds
1 tbsp ground flax seeds (linseed)

2 sheets dried nori, rolled and shredded
1 tbsp barley miso, mixed with 120ml warm water
50ml extra virgin olive or rapeseed oil

- Preheat the oven to 170°C/350°F/Gas Mark 4. Into a large bowl put the flour, black pepper, chia seeds, flax seeds and nori, and mix until combined.

- Pour in the miso mixture and mix together well, then with your hands start bringing it together as a dough. Trickle in the oil and continue to pull the mixture together. Sit it in a bowl and put in the fridge to chill for 20 minutes if you have time, or use straight away.

- Pull out the dough and roll into about 34 balls, then flatten each of them with your hands. Lay them on baking sheets lined with parchment paper then place in the oven and bake for 15–20 minutes or until crisp. Leave to cool, then remove from the paper. These will keep in a sealed container for up to 1 week.

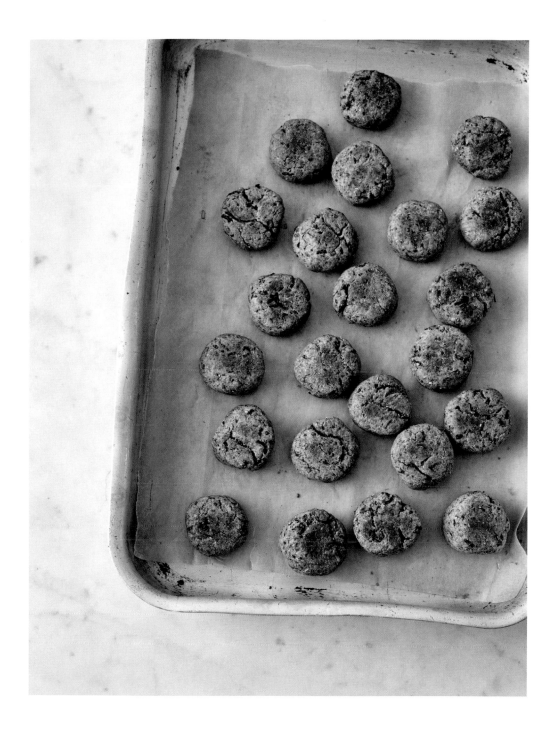

Caraway Oatcakes

Add a twist to regular oatcakes with the addition of caraway. I adore these for an afternoon snack, topped with a dab of almond butter or a small lump of cheese. Unpasteurised cheese is not recommended if you are pregnant or have a compromised immune system.

V MAKES 9–12   147–110 calories

200g medium organic oats or use fine oats if you prefer (you may need a little less water)
50g organic wholegrain spelt flour, plus extra for dusting
1 tsp bicarbonate of soda
2 tsp caraway seeds

Sea salt and freshly ground black pepper
50g organic butter, cubed
100ml warm water

Equipment: A 6cm round cutter

- Preheat the oven to 190°C/375°F/Gas Mark 5. Into a large bowl put the oats, flour, bicarbonate of soda and caraway seeds, then season well with the sea salt and freshly ground black pepper. Mix well.

- Add the butter and rub the mixture with your fingertips until it resembles breadcrumbs, then trickle in the water and knead until it comes together as a dough. Add more or less water, as needed.

- Dust a board with extra spelt flour and turn the dough out onto it. Dust a rolling pin, then roll out the mixture as thinly as you can. You will need to keep gathering and re-rolling as you go. Cut out as many rounds as you can (around 9–12, depending on thickness) and sit them on a baking sheet. Put in the oven and bake for about 20–25 minutes or until pale golden and firm. Remove and leave to cool. These will keep in a sealed container for up to 1 week.

Serve with ...

Unpasteurised blue cheese
Unpasteurised goat's cheese
Apple, celery or fennel slices

Top with ...
Asparagus Pâté (page 138)
Beetroot Dip (page 146)

Banana and Cinnamon Muffins

Who doesn't love muffins? But not if they're stuffed with refined sugar and unhealthy fats! By contrast, these hearty muffins are sweetened with the anti-inflammatory spice cinnamon, plus banana and apple. And if you wanted to up the protein content, you could always substitute half the flour for soya flour, or a vegan protein powder.

v MAKES 6   278 calories

125g organic wholegrain spelt flour   100ml extra virgin olive or rapeseed oil
1 tsp baking powder   100ml organic whole (full-fat) milk
1 tsp bicarbonate of soda   2 organic eggs
1–2 tsp ground cinnamon   1 eating apple, grated
¼ tsp freshly grated nutmeg   3 bananas, mashed

- Preheat the oven to 190°C/375°F/Gas Mark 5. Put the flour, baking powder, bicarbonate of soda, cinnamon and nutmeg into a large bowl.

- In another bowl put the oil, milk and eggs and beat together, then add the apple and bananas and mix. Tip into the flour mixture and gently beat together until combined. Do not over-beat – lumps are fine in muffin batter.

- Line a large 6-hole muffin tin with paper cases and spoon the mixture into each one. Place in the oven for 25–30 minutes or until risen and golden. Remove the muffins from the oven and transfer to a wire rack to cool. Best eaten on the day of baking.

Liz's Beauty Bombs

You may recognise these tasty and very more-ish skin-friendly snacks from my bestselling *Skin* book. Here I've developed a couple more tasty new versions, both enriched with the gut-healthy goodness of prebiotic ingredients. I truly love them!

Chocolate, Ginger and Matcha Bombs

 V DF GF **MAKES 18 SMALL BALLS**
PREP: OVERNIGHT SOAKING   *47 calories*

2 tsp pumpkin seeds, soaked overnight and ground
100g ground almonds
1 tsp good-quality matcha
2 tsp flax seeds, (linseed), ground
1 ball of stem ginger, roughly chopped
1 tbsp raw cacao powder
1–2 tsp raw or manuka honey

- Blitz the pumpkin seeds in a food processor until fine, then add the almonds, matcha, flax seeds and ginger and blitz again. Add the cacao and honey and whizz until combined, then add 2–4 tsp of warm water (1 tsp at a time) until it becomes a sticky dough. Go easy with the water as you don't want the bombs too wet.

- Remove from the food processor and transfer to a bowl. Cover and put in the fridge for 30 minutes to chill. Once firmed up, roll walnut-sized pieces into balls in your hands and sit them on a baking sheet lined with greaseproof paper, then put back in the fridge to firm up. Transfer to an airtight container – they will keep for up to 1 week.

Coconut Oat Bombs

 V DF **MAKES ABOUT 14 SMALL BALLS**   *44 calories*

30g pecan nuts, soaked overnight
30g medium oats
30g coconut pieces
100g prunes, roughly chopped
Pinch finely ground nutmeg

- Blitz the pecans, oats and coconut in a food processor until fine. Add the prunes and nutmeg and blitz again until well combined and the mixture comes together. Add 1 tsp of water if needed and whizz until it forms a dough.

- Transfer to a bowl, cover and chill for 30 minutes to firm up. Roll into walnut-sized balls, sit them on a baking sheet lined with greaseproof paper and return to the fridge to firm up. Transfer to an airtight container – they will keep for up to 1 week.

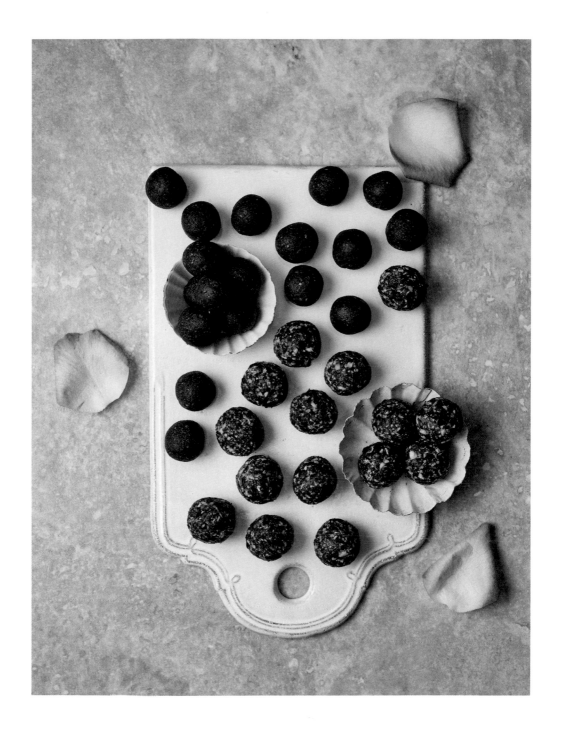

LIGHT MEALS

Turmeric Spiced Kedgeree

This is one of my favourite quick, yet filling, lunches. Again, it contains turmeric and garlic to bolster gut health, as well as parsley to help cleanse and detoxify the gut.

GF SERVES 4   491 calories

4 organic eggs

1 tbsp extra virgin olive or rapeseed oil

1 onion, finely chopped

Sea salt and freshly ground black pepper

3 cloves garlic, finely chopped

2 tsp turmeric

300g wholegrain basmati rice

900ml water

250g undyed smoked haddock fillets, skinned

100g frozen or fresh peas (soak frozen peas in boiling water for 1 minute and drain)

Handful of flat-leaf parsley, finely chopped

To serve:

Lemon wedges

4 tbsp plain Greek yoghurt

- Put the eggs in a pan of boiling water for 5 minutes, remove and immerse in cold water. Put to one side to cool. Heat the oil in a large lidded frying pan, add the onion and season well with the sea salt and freshly ground black pepper. Cook for a couple of minutes, then stir in the garlic and turmeric and cook for a few seconds more.

- Now tip in the rice and stir really well so it absorbs all the flavours. Pour in the water, turn the heat up a little and bring to the boil, then put the lid on and simmer for about 30 minutes or until the rice is tender and has absorbed all the water.

- While the rice is cooking, put the fish into another large frying pan, cover with water and simmer gently with the lid on for about 5 minutes or until the fish is opaque and almost cooked through. Remove with a fish slice, drain and flake into chunky pieces, then carefully stir it into the rice along with the peas. Taste, and season some more if needed.

- Transfer to serving plates, sprinkle with the parsley and garnish with the lemon wedges and peeled and quartered eggs. Serve with a tablespoon of yoghurt on the side of each plate.

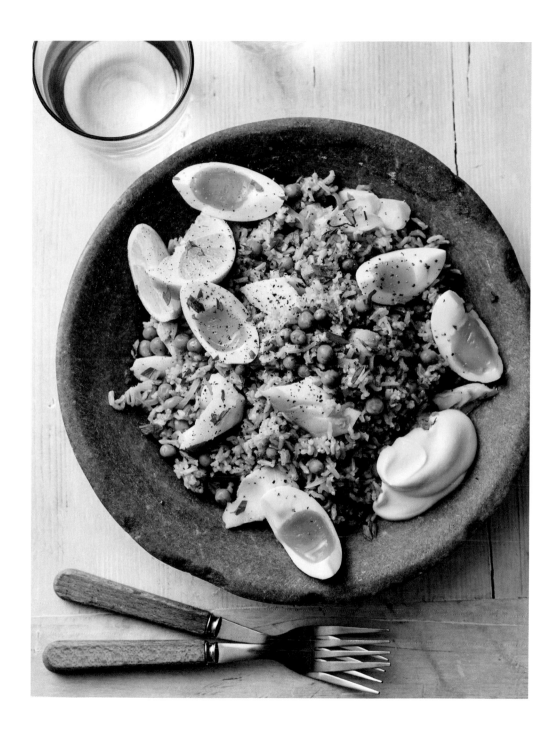

Jerusalem Artichoke Soup

When it comes to prebiotics, you can't beat Jerusalem artichokes and fennel, both of which star in this nourishing soup. For a more substantial meal, add a slice or two of homemade sourdough bread to serve alongside.

v SERVES 4   117 calories

1 tbsp extra virgin olive or rapeseed oil
1 onion, finely chopped
Sea salt and freshly ground black pepper
3 cloves garlic, finely chopped
3 sage leaves, chopped

500g Jerusalem artichokes, peeled and roughly chopped
½ fennel bulb, trimmed and finely chopped
900ml hot vegetable stock
4 tsp plain Greek yoghurt, to serve

- Heat the oil in a large pan, add the onion, season with the sea salt and freshly ground black pepper and cook for 2–3 minutes until beginning to soften. Stir through the garlic and sage and cook for a minute more, being careful the herbs don't catch and burn.

- Add the Jerusalem artichokes and the fennel, stir so everything gets coated and combined, then add a little of the stock. Raise the heat and let it bubble, add the remaining stock and bring to the boil, then reduce to a simmer and cook for about 20 minutes or until the artichokes are tender. Top up with hot water from the kettle if needed.

- Taste, and season some more if necessary. Then remove from the heat, ladle into a liquidiser a little at a time and blitz until smooth. Serve piping hot with a dollop of yoghurt on top.

Chicory and Roquefort Salad

This has to be one of the best gut-healing salads going, thanks to its prebiotic chicory, cleansing celery, digestion-boosting apple cider vinegar and the probiotic-rich Roquefort. Perfect as a starter, or just on its own in the summer.

GF SERVES 4
PREP: OVERNIGHT SOAKING   368 calories

4 red and white chicory bulbs (or just use one
    colour), trimmed and leaves separated
2 firm eating apples, sliced and tossed in lemon
    juice to prevent discoloration
1 stalk celery, finely chopped
100g Roquefort cheese, crumbled
Freshly ground black pepper
100g pecan nuts, soaked overnight in water, then
    drained
Small handful of flat-leaf parsley, finely chopped

For the dressing:
2 tbsp extra virgin olive oil
1 tbsp Apple Cider Vinegar (page 102)
    or Kombucha (page 104)
Sea salt and freshly ground black pepper

- First make the dressing. Put the oil into a small bowl or jug, add the apple cider vinegar or kombucha and sea salt and pepper and whisk until combined. Put to one side.

- Put the chicory leaves onto a large shallow platter, top with the apple, celery and Roquefort, season with a little freshly ground black pepper and scatter over the pecan nuts.

- When ready to serve, drizzle over the dressing and sprinkle with the parsley.

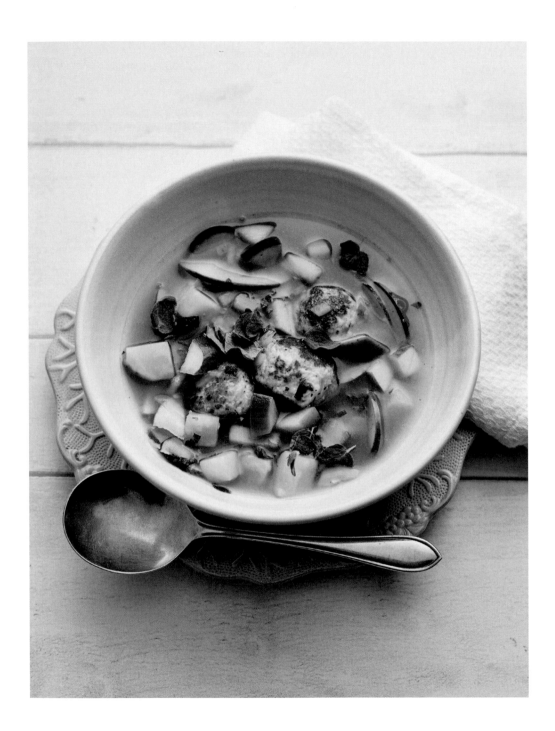

Broth with Chicken Meatballs, Celeriac and Apple

My family love this tasty, filling chicken meatball broth, plus the apple and celeriac give it a prebiotic boost. A wonderfully warming and nourishing dish.

DF SERVES 4 (MAKES 16 MEATBALLS)   272 calories

2 organic chicken breasts, skinned
Sea salt and freshly ground black pepper
1 onion, ½ roughly chopped, ½ finely chopped
Small handful of fresh oregano stalks, leaves only
2 tbsp olive or rapeseed oil

2 cloves garlic, finely chopped
1 celeriac (1kg), peeled and cubed
900ml organic chicken stock (see tip)
2 eating apples, roughly chopped

- Preheat the oven to 190°C/375°F/Gas Mark 5.

- Put the chicken, sea salt and pepper, roughly chopped onion and half the oregano into a food processor. Blitz until combined. Roll walnut-sized scoops of the mixture into balls. Put them on a baking sheet lined with parchment paper and chill for 20 minutes if time – if not, cook straight away.

- Put half the oil into a large frying pan and add the chicken balls – you may have to do this in two batches. Add a little more oil if needed. Cook on a medium heat for 3 minutes each side or until golden all over, remove with a slotted spoon and put on a plate lined with kitchen paper.

- Heat the remaining oil in a large lidded ovenproof cooking pot – a cast iron one is perfect. Add the finely chopped onion, season, and cook for 2–3 minutes until soft, then stir in the garlic. Cook for a few seconds, then add the celeriac and remaining oregano and cook for a further 5 minutes, moving it around the pan until it starts to colour. Pour in the chicken stock, bring to the boil, then reduce to a simmer. Add the chicken meatballs, put the lid on and put in the oven for 1½ hours, checking every half an hour or so to see if it needs topping up with hot water. Add the apples for the last 20 minutes of cooking. Remove from the oven, and ladle into shallow bowls to serve.

Superfood Sunshine Salad

It would be hard to pack more pre- and probiotic foods into a dish if you tried! The green veggies here feed our good-gut bugs, while cold potatoes are rich in resistant starch – much more so than hot ones. What's more, the apple cider vinegar or kombucha helps your stomach digest it all.

V GF **SERVES 4**   *272 calories*

1kg organic new potatoes
125g asparagus tips, trimmed
200g fresh or frozen peas
1 tbsp plain Greek yoghurt
Juice of ½ lemon
100g sugar snap peas, finely sliced
1 fennel bulb, trimmed and finely sliced and tossed
    in lemon juice to prevent discoloration
Sea salt and freshly ground black pepper
Pinch sumac (optional)
75g alfalfa sprouts (or sprout your own – mung
    beans and lentils are the easiest for beginners)

For the pickled radishes:
100g radishes, trimmed and finely sliced
A few fresh thyme leaves
2 tsp Apple Cider Vinegar (page 102)
    or Kombucha (page 104)
Sea salt and freshly ground black pepper

- Put the potatoes into a pan of salted water and cook for 15–20 minutes or until tender, drain and put to one side to cool. Put the asparagus tips into a steamer or sit them, covered, in a metal colander over a pan of simmering water for about 5 minutes or until tender. Remove and put to one side.

- If using frozen peas, put them into a bowl and cover with boiling water, leave for 3–4 minutes, then drain. Serve fresh peas raw or, if you prefer them cooked, simmer in boiling water for a couple of minutes, then drain.

- Now make the pickled radishes: put the radishes, thyme and apple cider vinegar or kombucha into a bowl, season with the sea salt and freshly ground black pepper and mix well, then put to one side.

- In another bowl mix the yoghurt and lemon juice together and season to taste. Set aside.

Into a large bowl put the peas, sugar snap peas and fennel, chop the asparagus and add, season lightly and toss together. Halve or quarter the cold potatoes and put onto a serving platter along with the pea and fennel mix. Then dot over the yoghurt, sprinkle with sumac (if using), and scatter over the alfalfa sprouts. Spoon the radish pickle onto the side of the platter or serve separately in a small bowl.

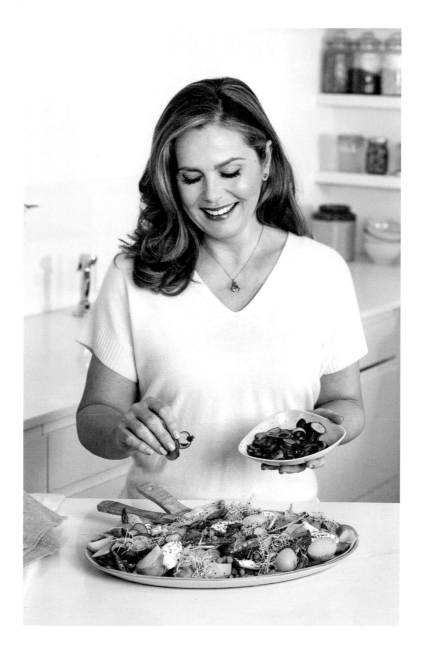

Superfood Cold Weather Salad

Who said salads need to be all about lettuce? This autumnal recipe is a mini-meal in itself. The butternut squash is packed with antioxidants, the gluten-free quinoa is rich in protein and the addition of nuts and seeds (you can soak them overnight) gives added gut-boosting benefits. Any leftovers can be refrigerated and eaten the next day.

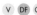 **SERVES 4**
PREP: OVERNIGHT SOAKING (OPTIONAL)   429 calories

---

1 butternut squash, halved, peeled and deseeded
1 tbsp extra virgin olive oil
Sea salt and freshly ground black pepper
Pinch ground cinnamon
180g quinoa
2–3 tsp Apple Cider Vinegar (page 102)
   or Kombucha (page 104)

200g spinach
1kg cooked fresh beetroots, roughly chopped
3 tsp pumpkin seeds
25g pecan nuts

• Preheat the oven to 200°C/400°F/Gas Mark 6. Put the squash into a roasting tin, add the olive oil, season with the sea salt and freshly ground black pepper and add the cinnamon. Using your hands, toss everything together. Put in the oven and roast for 20–30 minutes or until golden and tender. Remove and put to one side.

• While the squash is cooking, put the quinoa into a large lidded pan, cover with water so it sits halfway above the grains and season with sea salt. Cook on a low heat with the lid on for about 20 minutes. If it starts to dry out too much, top up with a little hot water. Remove from the heat, leaving the lid on, and put to one side for 10 minutes.

• Tip the quinoa into a large bowl, fluff up with a fork and add the apple cider vinegar or kombucha, season well and stir to combine. Stir in half the spinach, then transfer to a large shallow platter and top with the butternut squash, the remaining spinach and the beetroot. Scatter over the pumpkin seeds and nuts, to serve.

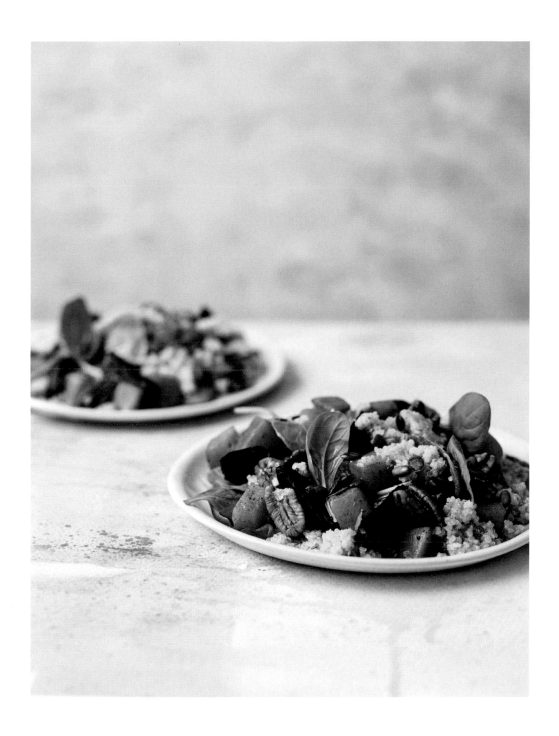

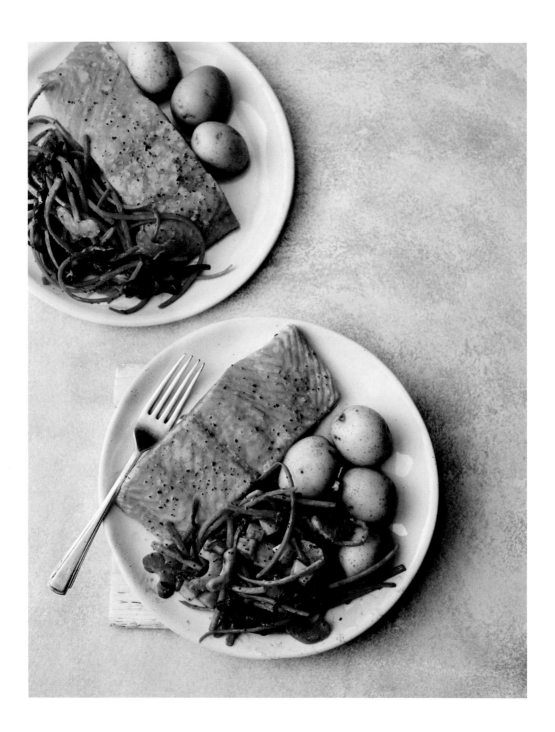

Mixed Slaw with Roasted Fish

The crunch of the slaw perfectly balances smooth, Omega-3-filled oily fish such as salmon and sardines. This is one of my favourite go-to lunch dishes.

GF SERVES 4   515 calories

4 × 150g fillets of wild salmon, or 8 fat sardines,
    skin on
1 tbsp olive or rapeseed oil
Sea salt and freshly ground black pepper
500g boiled organic new potatoes, served cold

For the slaw:
2 stalks celery, finely chopped
2 large carrots, peeled and grated
2 eating apples, cut into bite-size cubes
2 tbsp white or red Sauerkraut, or add 1 tbsp of
    each if you have (page 108)
2 tbsp plain Greek yoghurt
2 tsp poppy seeds

Preheat the oven to 190°C/375°F/Gas Mark 5. Sit the fish in a roasting tin, drizzle over the oil and season with the sea salt and freshly ground black pepper. Put in the oven and roast for 10–15 minutes or until cooked through. Remove and put to one side.

While the fish is cooking, prepare the slaw. Put the celery, carrots, apples and sauerkraut into a large bowl and stir. Add the yoghurt and stir again until well combined, then add the poppy seeds and give it one last stir. You probably don't need to season it as the sauerkraut is quite salty, but do taste and if you think it needs it, add just a little.

Transfer the roasted fish to serving plates along with a spoonful of slaw and serve with the cold new potatoes (a good source of bacteria-boosting resistant starch).

Miso and Ginger Squash Broth

When it comes to healing our gut, broth is one of our very best friends. The addition of medicinal mushrooms creates a meaty texture but also ramps up the immune-boosting potency of this great probiotic dish.

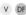 V DF SERVES 6   102 calories

1 tbsp extra virgin olive or rapeseed oil
1 onion, finely chopped
Sea salt and freshly ground black pepper
2 cloves garlic, finely chopped
5cm piece fresh ginger, peeled and grated or
    finely chopped
1 cinnamon stick, broken

2 sage leaves, chopped
1 small butternut squash, peeled, halved,
    deseeded and cubed
1 tbsp barley miso mixed with 1.1 litres warm
    water
200g shiitake mushrooms, large ones halved

- Heat the oil in a large lidded pan, add the onion and season with the sea salt and freshly ground black pepper. Cook for 3–4 minutes until the onion is soft, then stir in the garlic, ginger, cinnamon and sage and cook for a further minute.

- Add the squash and stir well so it soaks up all the flavours, cook for a few minutes, then add a little of the miso stock and let it bubble. Pour in the remaining miso, bring it to the boil, then reduce to a simmer. Put the lid on and let it cook gently for about 30 minutes, adding the shiitake mushrooms for the last 5 minutes of cooking.

- Taste, and season some more – it may need plenty of freshly ground black pepper. Ladle into bowls and enjoy piping hot.

LIZ'S TIP

If you like turmeric, this recipe also works well if you add a teaspoon of this super-spice alongside the other herbs and spices.

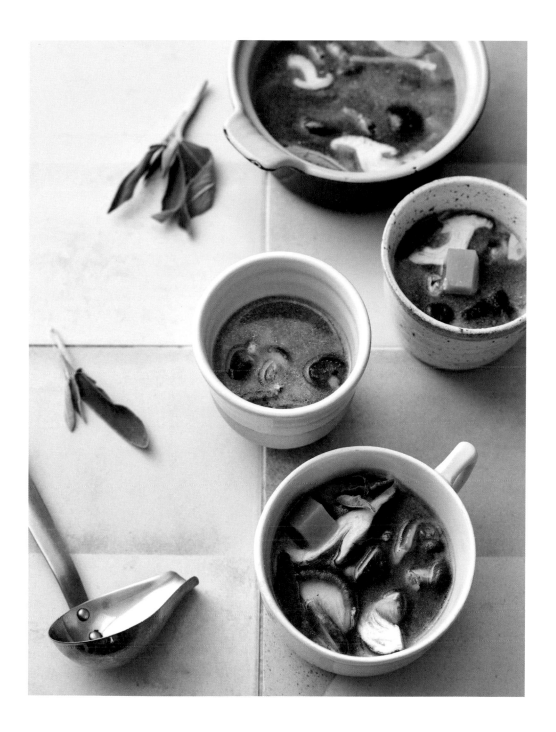

Deconstructed Sushi

Perhaps you thought carbs would be off the menu? But cooked and cooled sushi rice is high in resistant starch – like potatoes – so it can occasionally be a good addition when teamed with oily fish to lower the overall glycaemic load on our body.

 SERVES 4   365 calories

200g short-grain brown rice

Pinch sea salt

2 tsp rice vinegar

1 sheet dried nori, rolled and finely shredded

150g shiitake mushrooms, sliced

1 avocado, halved, stoned and sliced

2 tbsp red cabbage Sauerkraut (page 108; optional)

4 radishes, trimmed and very finely sliced

1 spring onion, trimmed and finely sliced

5cm piece cucumber, halved lengthways, seeds removed and sliced into strips

200g wild smoked salmon, roughly sliced (optional)

1 tsp pickled ginger

For the marinade:

1 tsp barley miso

2 tsp mirin (a rice wine)

2.5cm piece fresh ginger, peeled and grated

2 cloves garlic, grated or finely chopped

To serve:

Pinch black sesame seeds (optional)

Lime wedges (optional)

- Put the rice into a lidded pan and cover with twice the amount of water. Add a pinch of sea salt and cook with the lid on for about 30 minutes or until the rice is tender and the water has been absorbed. Tip the rice into a bowl and while still warm add the rice vinegar and the nori and mix well, then put to one side to cool.

- Mix the marinade ingredients together in a bowl, add the mushrooms and stir to coat.

- Heat a frying pan to hot. Put in the mushrooms and the marinade and cook, moving it all around the pan for a few minutes and letting the sauce bubble a little. Remove from the heat and leave to one side to cool.

- Assemble the serving bowls: spoon in the cooled rice, and add the avocado, sauerkraut, radishes, spring onion and cucumber. Then add the smoked salmon and pickled ginger and spoon on the mushrooms. Sprinkle with the black sesame seeds and a squeeze of lime (if using).

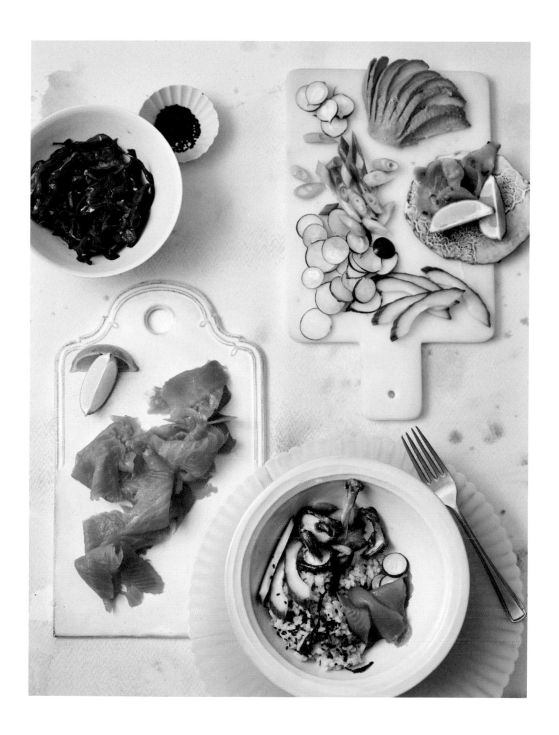

Quinoa Tabbouleh

Combining these tasty veg with zesty lemons and herbs creates a truly terrific taste sensation! This is a great meal in itself, or try serving alongside grilled meats or cheese at a summer barbecue.

V DF GF SERVES 4–6

PRESERVED LEMONS: MAKES A 1-LITRE JAR; PRESERVING TIME 6–8 WEEKS   326–217 calories

For the preserved lemons:
6 organic unwaxed lemons, quartered
4 tbsp sea salt
Juice of 4–5 lemons (enough to cover lemons)

For the tabbouleh:
300g carrots, peeled and sliced lengthways
1 fennel bulb, trimmed and roughly chopped
1 tbsp extra virgin olive or rapeseed oil
Sea salt and freshly ground black pepper
300g quinoa
Handful of mint leaves, finely chopped
Handful of flat-leaf parsley, finely chopped

- To preserve the lemons, put the lemon quarters into a 1-litre sterilised sealable jar, shaking in the salt as you go. Pour in the lemon juice to cover, and press it all down so it's tightly packed. Secure with the lid and set aside for 6–8 weeks.

- To make the tabbouleh, preheat the oven to 200°C/400°F/Gas Mark 6. Put the carrots and fennel into a roasting tin, drizzle over the oil and season with the sea salt and freshly ground black pepper. Toss it all together with your hands and put it in the oven for about 20–30 minutes, or until the vegetables are tender. Remove from the oven and, when cool enough to handle, chop into strips.

- While the vegetables are roasting, put the quinoa into a lidded pan and cover with twice the amount of water. Add a pinch of salt and cook with the lid on for about 20 minutes or until the quinoa is cooked and has absorbed all the water. Remove the pan from the heat and, leaving the lid on, put it to one side for 5–10 minutes, then fluff up with a fork.

- Transfer to a large bowl, then add the roasted vegetables and herbs and season well. Serve with the homemade preserved lemons or use bought ones.

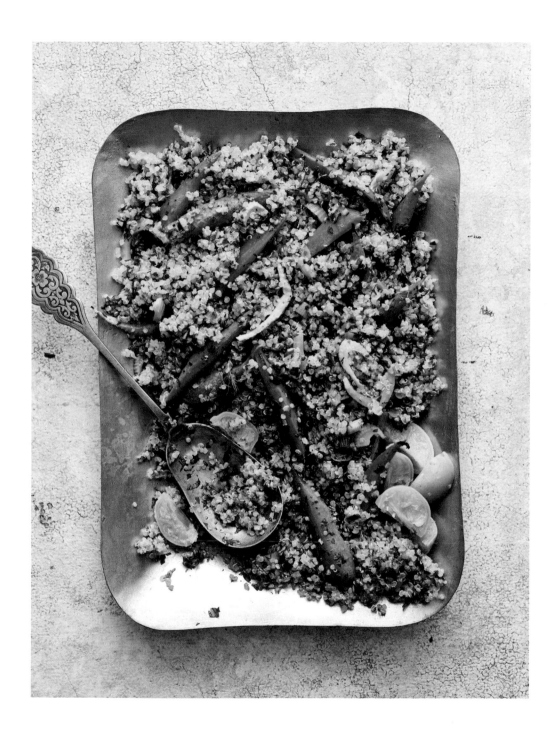

Miso Stir-fry

Quick, easy and super-friendly to our gut, this stir-fry is pretty foolproof. Perfect for a midweek meal when time is tight.

V DF SERVES 4   142 calories

1 tbsp sesame oil
3 spring onions, trimmed and finely chopped
5cm piece fresh ginger, grated or finely chopped
200g asparagus tips, trimmed and chopped into
    3cm pieces
Sea salt and freshly ground black pepper
250g pak choi, trimmed, leaves separated and
    sliced lengthways
125g shiitake mushrooms, large ones halved
300g straight-to-wok rice noodles

For the sauce:
1 tbsp barley miso
1 tbsp warm water
Juice of ½ orange
1 tsp low-salt tamari sauce

- Heat the oil in a large wok, add the spring onions and move them around the pan for a few seconds, then add the ginger and asparagus and cook for 3–4 minutes. Season with the salt and pepper.

- Add the pak choi and mushrooms to the wok and continue moving everything around, then cook for a few minutes until the vegetables start to soften a little.

- Now make the sauce. In a bowl mix the miso, water, orange juice and tamari. Push the vegetables to one side of the wok and add the sauce. Let it bubble for a while, then combine.

- Throw in the noodles and toss really well to heat through and so that everything gets well coated. Season with pepper and serve up.

LIZ'S TIP

A handy kitchen-cupboard ingredient, tamari is a gluten-free type of soy sauce. I prefer the lower-salt organic versions.

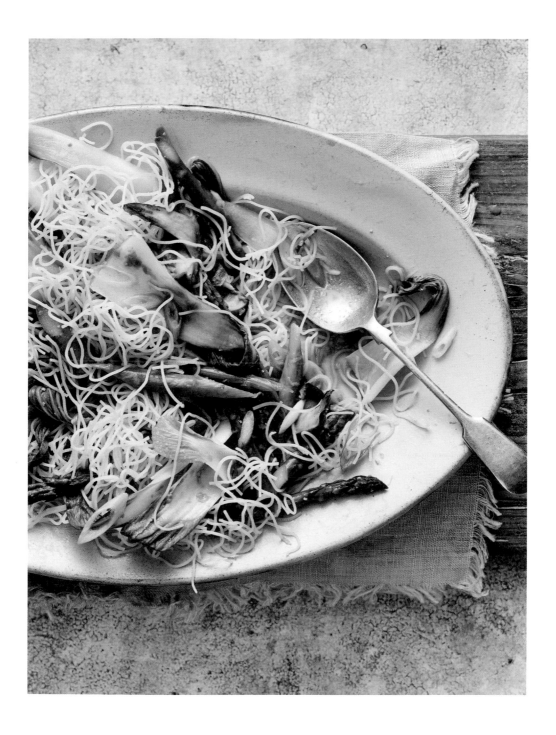

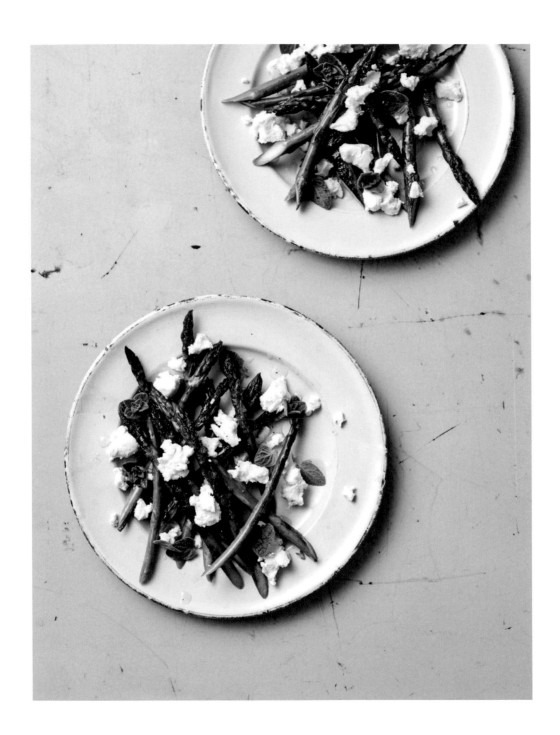

Chargrilled Asparagus with Goat's Cheese

Sometimes simplicity is best, with just one or two good-quality ingredients prepared perfectly to showcase their flavour. That's exactly what you get with these asparagus tips topped with goat's cheese, brought together with an even simpler dressing. Truly delicious.

V GF SERVES 6   320 calories

300g asparagus tips, trimmed
1 tbsp extra virgin olive oil
Sea salt and freshly ground black pepper
250g soft unpasteurised goat's cheese, crumbled
A few oregano leaves for garnish (and gut)

For the dressing:
3 tbsp extra virgin olive oil
1 tbsp Apple Cider Vinegar (page 102)
  or Kombucha (page 104)
Sea salt and freshly ground black pepper

- For the dressing, put the oil and apple cider vinegar or kombucha into a small bowl or jug, season well and whisk. Taste, adjust the seasoning if needed, and put to one side. Heat a griddle pan to hot, meanwhile tossing the asparagus with the olive oil and sea salt and freshly ground black pepper.

- Put the asparagus tips into the hot griddle pan and leave them undisturbed for about 3 minutes or until the underside is starting to char, then turn and cook the other side for about the same time or until the asparagus is tender. Transfer to a serving plate.

- Drizzle over half the dressing, then top with the goat's cheese and oregano. To serve, add the remaining dressing.

Marinated Tempeh with Avocado and Almonds

Tempeh and avocado are naturally squishy, so the addition of almonds makes for a nice crunchy contrast. Honey and orange sweeten the dish, while the low-salt tamari sauce adds an umami kick, so you're satisfying many tastebuds.

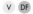 SERVES 4
PREP: OVERNIGHT CHILLING (IF TIME)   598 calories

240g (2 × 120g packs) tempeh, cut into cubes
1 tbsp olive or rapeseed oil
1 red onion, roughly chopped
200g spinach
2 avocados, halved, stoned and sliced
2 oranges, segmented
100g almonds, soaked (skinless are easier to digest)

For the dressing:
3 tbsp extra virgin olive oil
1 tbsp raspberry vinegar

For the marinade:
2 tbsp tamari sauce
Juice of ½ orange
1 tsp raw honey
A few thyme leaves
Freshly ground black pepper

- First make the marinade. Put the tamari, orange juice, honey and thyme leaves into a bowl and whisk together. Season with the freshly ground black pepper, then add the tempeh cubes and toss well. Cover and put in the fridge for an hour or so, or overnight if you have time.

- Make the dressing, mixing together the oil and vinegar. Season and put to one side.

- Heat the oil in a large frying pan, add the marinated tempeh and cook for about 5 minutes or until beginning to turn golden. Remove and put to one side, then add the onion to the pan and cook until softened, about 5 minutes. Add a trickle more oil if needed. Remove the onion and set aside, then put in the spinach and stir it around the pan until it just starts to wilt. Then transfer it to a serving plate or bowl.

- Top with the tempeh and onions, then add the avocado, orange segments and almonds. To serve, trickle over the dressing.

I first discovered tempeh, popular with vegans, back in the 1980s when I was a practising macrobiotic. Made with fermented soya beans solidified into a handy slab, it's a good meat alternative as well as being a very gut-friendly form of good-quality protein. A vacuum pack of tempeh will last for many weeks in the fridge and is useful for serving to vegans.

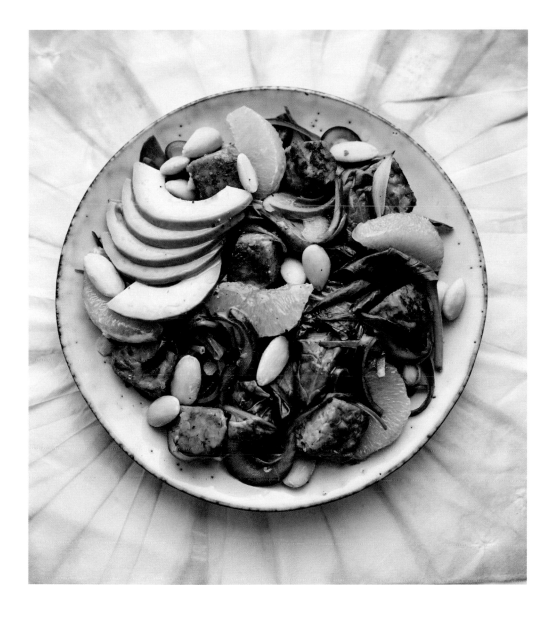

Haddock with Beetroot Salad

Fennel and fish work so well together. This dish takes a while to make so it's best suited to a weekend when you've got a little more time.

GF **SERVES 4**   226 calories

600g haddock (4 fillets) or similar, skinned
2 tsp fennel seeds, crushed
Sea salt and freshly ground black pepper
300ml organic milk
25g organic butter
1 onion, sliced
2 cloves garlic, finely sliced
200g organic or homegrown spinach
A few parsley stalks, leaves only, finely chopped

For the beetroot salad:
1kg raw beetroots, stalks trimmed
1 tbsp Apple Cider Vinegar (page 102)
   or Kombucha (page 104)
A few dill leaves, finely chopped

- First make the beetroot salad. Preheat the oven to 200°C/400°F/Gas Mark 6. Put the beetroots into a roasting tin, cover with water to halfway up the tin, then cover with foil. Put in the oven and cook for 1 hour, or until the beetroots are tender when poked with a sharp knife. Remove from the oven and the tin and put to one side until cool enough to peel. When cool, trim and remove the skins and slice the beetroots into sticks, put into a bowl with the apple cider vinegar or kombucha and the dill and turn to coat. Put to one side.

- Smother the haddock with the crushed fennel seeds and sea salt and pepper. Sit it in a large lidded frying pan and pour over the milk. Put the lid on and simmer gently for about 8–10 minutes or until the fish is opaque and cooked. Remove with a fish slice and set aside. (Don't throw away the milk.)

- While the fish is cooking, put the butter into another frying pan. When melted, add the onion and garlic, season well and cook for about 5 minutes or until softened, then add a ladle or two of the milk and whisk together in the pan. Throw in the spinach and stir until wilted.

- Divide the spinach and any sauce between four serving plates and add the haddock fillets, then sprinkle over the parsley. Spoon on the beetroot salad or serve on the side.

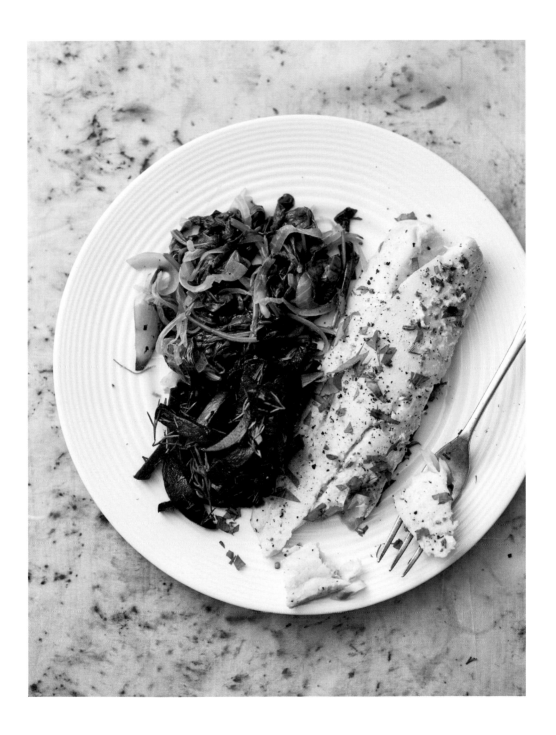

MAIN MEALS

Carrot Burgers with Apple Pickle

I love making burgers from all sorts of ingredients. My five children of all ages love this super-healthy veggie version and I like to serve with some steamed greens topped with the apple pickle.

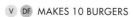 **MAKES 10 BURGERS**   112 calories (burger only)

1 tsp caraway seeds

1kg carrots, peeled and half roughly grated, half chopped

400g can butter beans, drained and rinsed

2 cloves garlic, roughly chopped

1 apple, roughly chopped

1 tbsp ground flax seeds (linseed)

Sea salt and freshly ground black pepper

1 organic egg, lightly beaten

1 tbsp olive or rapeseed oil, to fry

Toasted wholemeal or sourdough bread rolls, to serve

For the apple pickle:

2 eating apples, finely sliced

1 tbsp Apple Cider Vinegar (page 102) or Kombucha (page 104)

5cm piece fresh ginger, peeled and finely chopped

Sea salt and freshly ground black pepper

Handful of flat-leaf parsley, leaves only, finely chopped

- Put the caraway seeds into a food processor and blitz until crushed, then add the chopped carrots, butter beans, garlic, apple and flax seeds and season well. Whizz until really well mixed, add the egg and mix again, then tip out into a large bowl and mix in the grated carrot.

- Divide into 10 large balls, roll and then sit them on a baking sheet lined with greaseproof paper. Put in the fridge to chill for 20 minutes.

- To make the apple pickle, put the apples, vinegar and ginger into a bowl, season well and stir. Taste, and adjust the seasoning if necessary, then stir in the parsley and put to one side.

- Remove the carrot balls from the fridge, pat them down with the flat of your hand to make the burgers. Heat the olive oil in a large non-stick frying pan and put in a few burgers at a time. Cook on a low heat until the undersides are golden – this will take about 10 minutes, so don't cook on a high heat or they'll burn. When they feel a bit more stable, with a fish slice carefully turn them over and cook the other side for about the same time. Continue cooking all the burgers (you can freeze any leftover ones).

- Serve sandwiched in the toasted rolls with some apple pickle.

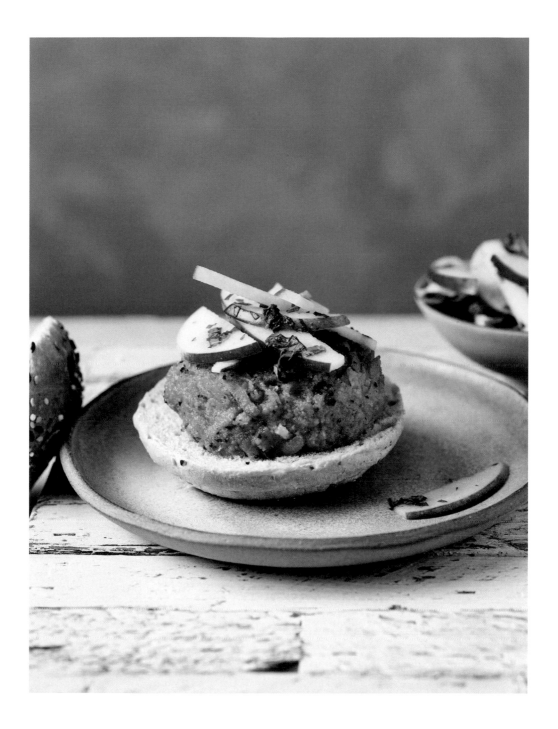

Beef Broth Casserole

Slow-cooked stews make filling meals that are easy on our digestion, as all the ingredients have had time to soften. Good to make over a weekend – and once you've made a batch of broth you can freeze any you don't need right away and use another time, for so many other recipes (or simply enjoy drinking it neat).

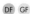 **DF** **GF** **SERVES 4**

PREP: ABOUT 6 HOURS FOR THE BROTH, CASSEROLE COOKING TIME 3–4 HOURS   354 calories

900ml Beef Bone Broth (page 66)

2 tbsp olive or rapeseed oil

600g grass-fed shin or skirt of beef, cut into chunky pieces

Sea salt and freshly ground black pepper

1 onion, finely chopped

2 stalks celery, finely chopped

1 bay leaf

4 sage leaves, finely chopped

4 large carrots, peeled and roughly chopped

2 leeks (250g), trimmed and roughly chopped

120g shiitake mushrooms, large ones halved

Handful of steamed greens, to serve

- First make the broth following the recipe on page 66.

- When you're ready to make the casserole, preheat the oven to 170°C/350°F/Gas Mark 4. Heat half the oil in a large lidded cast-iron casserole pot, add the beef and season with the sea salt and freshly ground black pepper. You may need to do this in batches, or you'll overcrowd the pot and steam the beef rather than brown it. Cook until browned all over, then remove and put to one side. Put in the remaining oil and the onion, cook for a couple of minutes, then add the celery, bay leaf and sage and cook for a further 4 minutes or until soft. Pour in a little broth and stir to dislodge any bits from the bottom of the pot to deglaze it. Let it bubble, then add the remaining broth and bubble for a few more minutes. Reduce the heat and return the meat to the pot. Cover and put in the oven for 1½–2 hours.

- Remove from the oven and add the carrots and leeks, stir and top up with a little hot water if needed, then put back in the oven and cook for a further hour or until the vegetables are tender and the meat is tender enough for you to cut through it with a spoon. Tip in the mushrooms for the last 20 minutes of cooking.

- Remove from the oven, taste, and season some more if needed. Ladle into bowls and serve piping hot with some seasonal steamed greens.

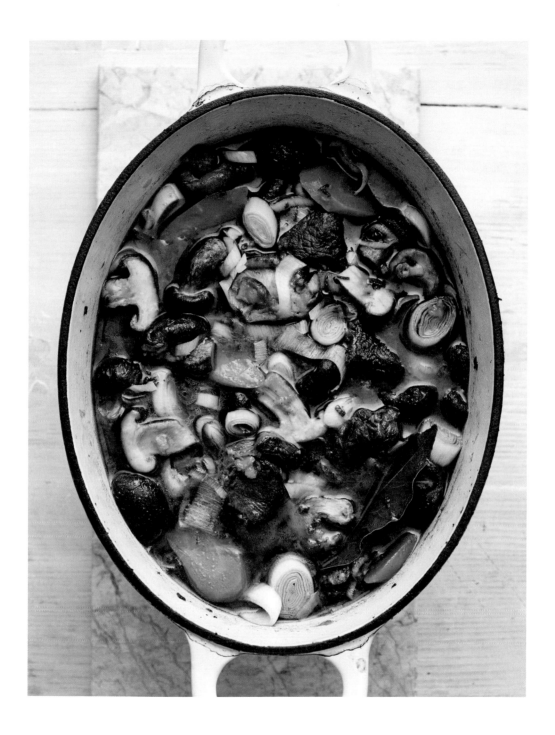

Squash and Spinach Curry

As I mentioned earlier, if you're still not a convert to the tangy taste of kimchi, you can hide it in other dishes! This vegetarian curry has not only a generous helping of probiotic-packed kimchi added in, but also plenty of herbs and spices to kick-start our metabolism (just omit the chilli if you're sensitive to them, or prefer this less hot).

V SERVES 4   576 calories

1 butternut squash, halved, peeled, deseeded and cubed

2 tbsp extra virgin olive oil

Sea salt and freshly ground black pepper

1 onion, finely chopped

2 cloves garlic, finely chopped

1 red chilli, deseeded and finely chopped (optional)

5cm piece fresh ginger, peeled and finely chopped

1 tbsp garam masala

2 tsp turmeric

1 tsp coriander seeds, ground

1 tsp ground fenugreek

1 tbsp tomato purée

125g ground almonds (preferably home-ground, skins and all)

500ml hot vegetable stock

400ml can coconut milk

200g spinach

1–2 tbsp homemade Kimchi (page 110), chopped

For the raita:

4–5 tbsp plain Greek yoghurt

½ cucumber, peeled, halved lengthways, deseeded and finely chopped

Small handful of fresh mint leaves, finely chopped

Sea salt and freshly ground black pepper

- Preheat the oven to 200°C/400°F/Gas Mark 6. Put the squash into a roasting tin, add half the oil and season with the sea salt and freshly ground black pepper. Toss together with your hands, then put it in the oven and roast for about 20–30 minutes until golden and tender. Remove and put to one side.

- While the squash is cooking, heat the remaining oil in a large heavy-based lidded pan, add the onion and cook for 2–3 minutes and season well, then throw in the garlic and cook for a further few seconds. Stir in the chilli (if using), ginger, garam masala, turmeric, coriander and fenugreek and cook for a few more minutes, then stir through the tomato purée. Tip in the ground almonds and stir really well, so everything gets completely coated.

- Now pour in the stock and coconut milk, and on a low heat stir well until smooth. Cook on a low simmer with the lid on for about 20–30 minutes, topping up with a little hot water as it starts to thicken. Taste, and adjust the seasoning as needed, then throw in the roasted squash and the spinach and stir until the spinach has wilted. Stir in the kimchi and heat through for just a few seconds, then remove the pan from the heat.

- While the curry is cooking prepare the raita. Mix together the yoghurt, cucumber and fresh mint and season to taste. Serve alongside the curry.

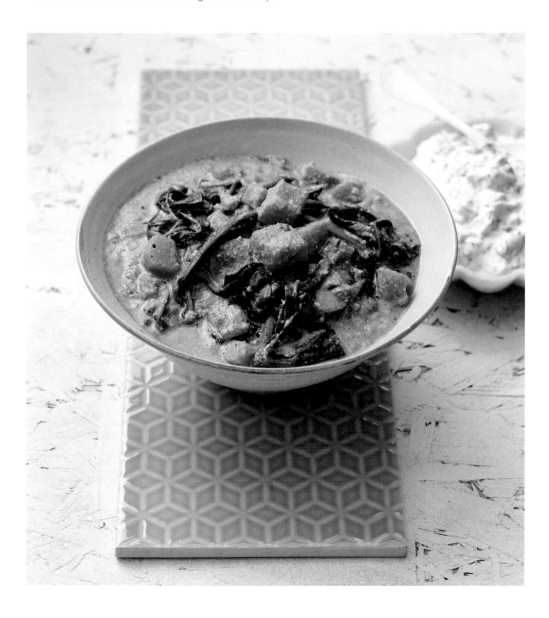

Duck with Miso, Wild Rice and Red Cabbage Sauerkraut

I've become slightly obsessed with Carmague red rice ever since I discovered it's a fabulous source of B vitamins. These are often depleted when we're chronically stressed or have gut problems and aren't properly absorbing other nutrients. This rich red recipe helps boost our levels back up in the most delicious way.

DF SERVES 4   671 calories

300g red Camargue and wild rice (or other)
Sea salt and freshly ground black pepper
1 tsp miso mixed with 1 tsp warm water
2 oranges, segmented
4 duck breasts, skin on (about 800g total), scored
  in a criss-cross pattern with a sharp knife

Drizzle of olive or rapeseed oil
4 cloves garlic, skin on
2 eating apples, roughly chopped
A few stalks thyme, leaves only
4 tbsp red cabbage Sauerkraut (page 108)

- Put the rice into a large pan, cover with plenty of water – at least twice the amount of rice – add a pinch of the sea salt, cover and cook on a simmer for about 30 minutes or until the rice is tender. Remove from the heat and drain, return to the pan, stir in the miso mixture and orange segments and season with freshly ground black pepper. Put to one side.

- While the rice is cooking, preheat the oven to 190°C/375°F/Gas Mark 5. Season the duck breasts with the sea salt and freshly ground black pepper. Heat the oil in a large frying pan and add the duck breasts, skin side down. Cook on a medium heat for 10 minutes, then remove and transfer them to a roasting tin, skin side up. Add a tiny amount of oil along with the garlic and apple pieces and sprinkle on the thyme. Put in the oven and cook for a further 10 minutes.

- Remove the duck from the oven and let it sit for about 5 minutes, then slice it on the diagonal. Serve it with the roasted apples and garlic on a bed of wild rice, and a tablespoon of red cabbage sauerkraut on the side.

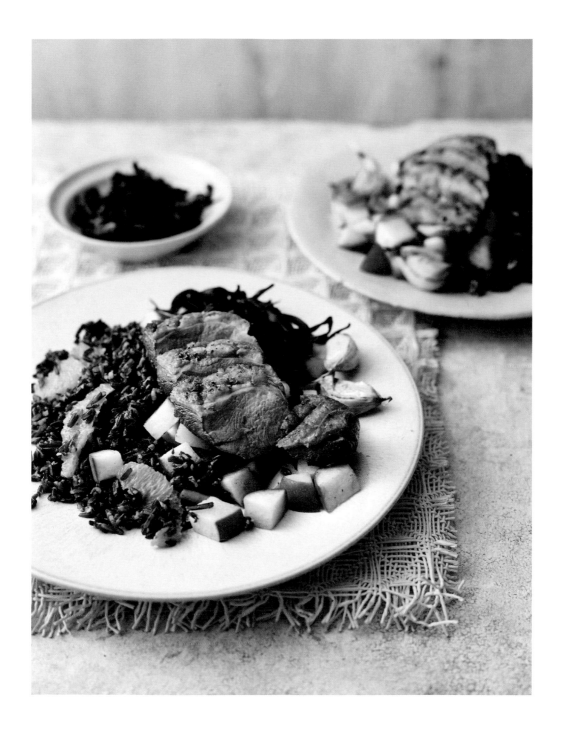

Chunky Fish Broth

Broths don't need to be meat-based. The bones of fish also make an excellent collagen-rich base to soothe our gut, plus the herbs in this recipe give it extra healing powers.

 SERVES 4   354 calories

1 tbsp olive or rapeseed oil
1 onion, roughly chopped
Sea salt and freshly ground black pepper
2 cloves garlic, roughly chopped
1 tsp fennel seeds, ground in a pestle and mortar
Pinch dried oregano
Pinch paprika
2 stalks celery, finely chopped
2 carrots, peeled and finely chopped
1 fennel bulb, trimmed, finely chopped (reserve fronds)
1 tbsp tomato purée
200g haddock loin, skinned, roughly chopped

200g monkfish tail, fine film removed, roughly chopped
200g hake, skinned, roughly chopped
Handful of flat-leaf parsley, finely chopped

For the stock:
2–3 fish heads from white fish (your fishmonger should give you these for free)
1 bay leaf
2 carrots, peeled and roughly chopped
1 onion, quartered
Sea salt and freshly ground black pepper

- First make the stock. Put the fish heads, bay leaf, carrots and onion into a large stockpot, cover with water to near the top of the pot and season with the sea salt and freshly ground black pepper. Bring to the boil, then reduce to a simmer, put the lid on and cook for 1 hour. Sieve into a large bowl or jug. Ideally you need about 1.7 litres of stock – freeze any leftovers.

- Heat the olive oil in a large lidded pan, add the onion, season well and cook for 3–4 minutes until softened. Stir through the garlic and cook for a few seconds, then add the fennel seeds, oregano and paprika and cook for a minute more. Add the celery, carrots and fennel and stir again. Cook on a low heat, stirring occasionally, for about 10 minutes or until the carrots begin to soften.

- Stir in the tomato purée, cook for a few seconds, then add a little of the fish stock and let it bubble. Add the remaining stock, bring to the boil, then put the lid on and simmer for 1 hour.

- Add the fish, cover and simmer for about 8 minutes or until the fish is cooked through. Be careful not to overcook it, though. Carefully stir in half the parsley, then ladle into soup bowls and sprinkle the rest on, to serve. Garnish with the reserved fennel fronds.

Griddled Turkey with Leek and Blue Cheese Gratin

Meat topped with delicious creamy cheese then sprinkled with a layer of toasty, crunchy breadcrumbs is a winning recipe in my book, especially when the meat is lean turkey, rich in tryptophan. Try this for a Saturday-night sofa supper.

SERVES 4   656 calories

4 organic turkey breasts
Drizzle of olive or rapeseed oil
Sea salt and freshly ground black pepper
A few thyme stalks, leaves only

For the gratin:
1 tbsp olive or rapeseed oil
20g organic butter
1 onion, finely chopped
Sea salt and freshly ground black pepper

2 cloves garlic, finely chopped
1 bay leaf
A few thyme stalks, leaves only
2 large leeks (about 800g)
200ml hot vegetable stock
100ml double cream
Pinch freshly grated nutmeg
125g Stilton or other blue cheese, crumbled
100g sourdough breadcrumbs

- Preheat the oven to 190°C/375°F/Gas Mark 5. First make the gratin: heat the oil and butter in a large pan, add the onion and season with the sea salt and freshly ground black pepper. Cook for 3–4 minutes until softened, then stir through the garlic and cook for a few more seconds. Add the bay, thyme and leeks and cook for about 6 minutes or until the leeks are just tender.

- Stir in the stock and cream and simmer for a couple of minutes, then transfer it all to an ovenproof dish. Remove the bay leaf and sprinkle over the nutmeg and dot over the cheese.

- Sprinkle over the breadcrumbs and put in the oven for 25–30 minutes until golden and bubbling. Remove and put to one side.

- While that's in the oven, cook the turkey breasts. Lay each one out between two sheets of cling film and bash with the edge of a rolling pin to flatten a little. Then rub them with the oil, season well and sprinkle over the thyme leaves. Heat a griddle pan to hot, add the turkey breasts, one or two at a time, and cook for about 4 minutes or until the undersides are beginning to char and each breast lifts away easily from the pan. Turn and cook the other side for the same time or until it's cooked through.

- Continue to cook all the turkey, then serve with the gratin.

All-in-One Roast Chicken

Tray bakes are just brilliant for those with large families like me, or who always have lots going on (ditto). Just throw all these fabulous ingredients into one large pan and go! You do need to add the leeks and artichokes later on with this one, but it's still oh-so-easy (like a Sunday morning . . .) and is a favourite family weekend staple.

DF **GF** **SERVES 4**   613 calories

1 organic chicken, cut into 4 (ask your butcher to do this, or use poultry shears), or 8 chicken thighs with bone in, skin on
1 bulb garlic, separated into cloves, skin left on
900g potatoes, peeled and quartered
2 tbsp olive or rapeseed oil

A few sage leaves, roughly chopped
Sea salt and freshly ground black pepper
500g Jerusalem artichokes, peeled or scrubbed and roughly chopped
3 leeks, trimmed and roughly chopped
Handful of flat-leaf parsley, finely chopped

- Preheat the oven to 200°C/400°F/Gas Mark 6. Put the chicken pieces into a large roasting tin along with the garlic and potatoes, drizzle over half the olive oil, add the sage and season well with the sea salt and freshly ground black pepper. Turn everything so it all gets coated. Put in the oven to roast for 1 hour or until the chicken is cooked through.

- Toss the Jerusalem artichokes and the leeks with the remaining oil, season, and add to the roasting tin, tucking them in and around the chicken and potatoes for the last 30 minutes of cooking. Remove from the oven and throw the parsley all over. To make this dish even easier, you can serve the tin straight to table.

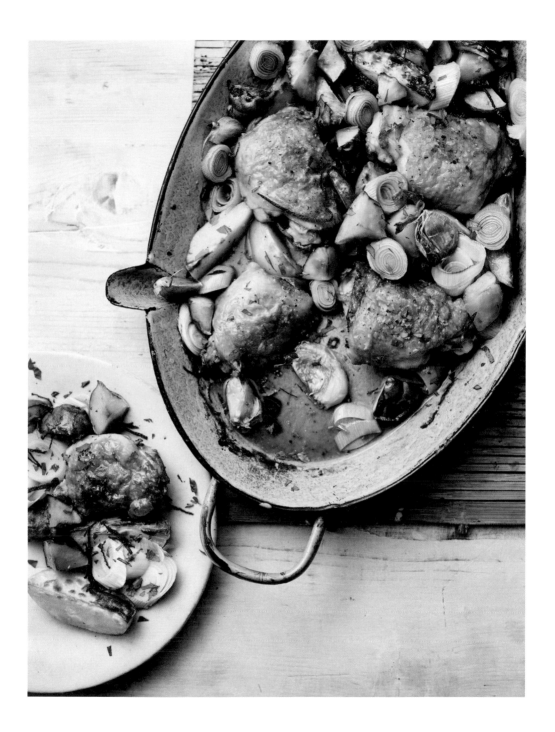

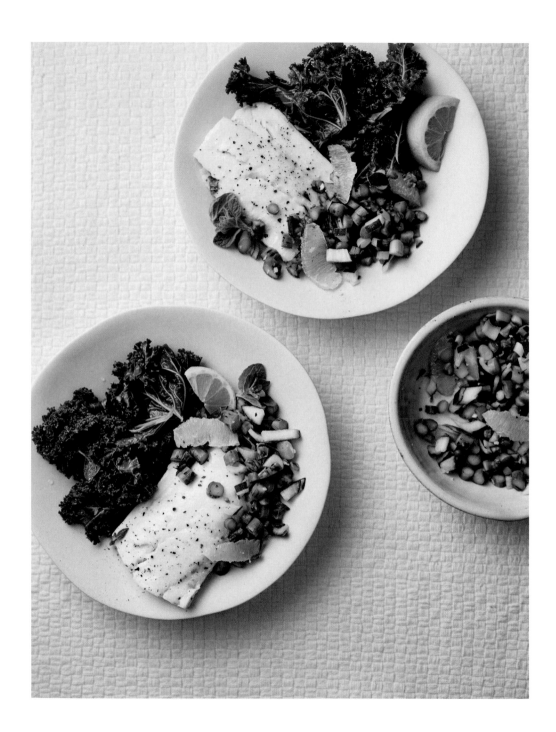

Ginger Poached Fish

I've tended to fry my fish for speed, but it's actually just as quick (if not quicker) to poach, and there's no need to worry about burning the skin or drying out the flesh. The salsa in this dish adds a lovely depth of flavour and a prebiotic punch.

 DF GF SERVES 4   190 calories

600g haddock loin (or similar), skinned and cut
    into 4 pieces
Sea salt and freshly ground black pepper
3 cloves garlic, finely sliced
A few oregano stalks, plus extra for garnish
5cm piece fresh ginger, peeled and finely sliced

For the asparagus salsa:
200g asparagus tips, trimmed
3 spring onions, trimmed
Drizzle of extra virgin olive oil
Sea salt and freshly ground black pepper
½ red onion, trimmed, soaked in water for
    10 minutes, then drained and chopped
1 clove garlic, finely chopped
1 lemon, segmented

To serve:
200g kale leaves, steamed and tossed with lemon
    juice
Lemon wedges

- First make the asparagus salsa. Heat a griddle pan to hot, toss the asparagus and spring onions with the olive oil and season well. Put them in the hot griddle pan and cook for about 2–3 minutes or until beginning to char, then turn using metal tongs and cook the other side for the same time. Remove, and when cool enough to handle, chop finely and transfer to a bowl. Add the red onion, garlic and lemon and stir together until well combined. Taste, season if required, and put to one side.

- Add the fish to a large lidded frying pan and cover with water, season and add the garlic, oregano and ginger. Put the lid on and simmer on low for about 8–10 minutes or until the fish is opaque and cooked through.

- Remove the fish pieces with a fish slice and transfer to serving plates. Serve with the steamed kale and the asparagus salsa on the side, and garnish with oregano and lemon wedges.

Roast Lamb with Garlic Crushed New Potatoes

My family are 100 per cent grass-fed livestock farmers (lamb and Hereford beef), so roast lamb is a tasty favourite in my house and the addition of crushed garlic and fennel ramps up the digestion-boosting factor. If you have any leftover potatoes from this dish, eat them cold tomorrow, sprinkled with a few spices for a gut-boosting prebiotic snack.

DF **GF** SERVES 4, PLUS LEFTOVERS   694 calories

Leg of grass-fed lamb, about 2kg
2 fennel bulbs, trimmed and roughly chopped
    (tossed in a little olive oil)
2 bulbs garlic, left whole and tops sliced off
Sea salt and freshly ground black pepper
Drizzle of olive or rapeseed oil
Handful of oregano leaves, roughly chopped

Handful of mint leaves, roughly chopped
Pinch sumac
1 tsp dried oregano
900g organic new potatoes
1 tbsp extra virgin olive oil
Steamed greens or asparagus to serve

- Preheat the oven to 220°C/425°F/Gas Mark 7. Sit the lamb, fennel and garlic in a large roasting tin and season well with sea salt and freshly ground black pepper. In a bowl put the olive oil, oregano, mint, sumac and dried oregano and mix together. Smother evenly all over the lamb. Put in the oven and cook for half an hour, then turn the oven down to 200°C/400°F/Gas Mark 6 and cook for a further hour. If you like your lamb pink, cook for a little less. Remove from the oven, cover with foil to keep warm and let it sit for about 20 minutes.

- While the lamb is cooking, put the potatoes in a pan of salted water, cook for about 15–20 minutes or until tender when poked with a sharp knife. Drain and return to the pan, add the extra virgin olive oil and squeeze the garlic out of several of the roasted garlic cloves onto the potatoes, then roughly crush them with the back of a fork. Taste, and season if required.

- Slice the lamb to serve, accompanied by the fennel, the crushed potatoes, any extra garlic cloves and some steamed greens or asparagus.

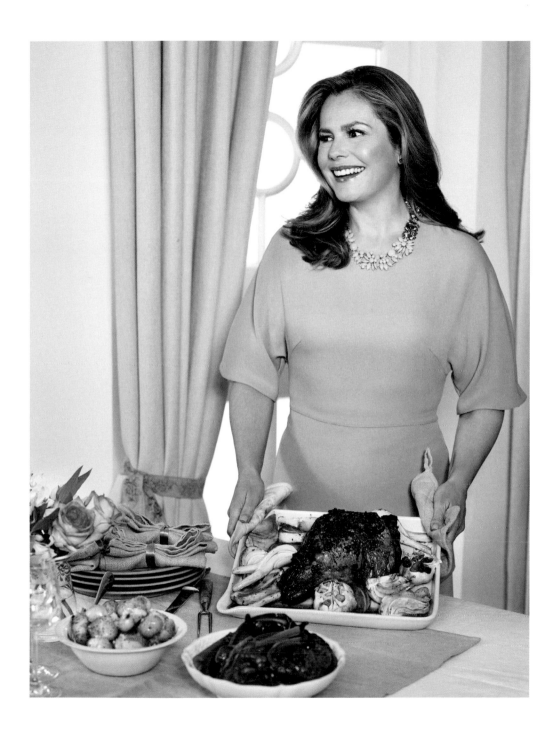

Black Bean Beef Short Ribs

Slow-cooking a stew helps break down all the lovely ingredients and makes it easier on our digestion. My older children, especially, love this hearty recipe for a warming winter dinner – but it's also great all year round.

 SERVES 4–6   645–430 calories

2kg short ribs (also called 'Jacob's Ladder') – you may need to pre-order from your butcher
Drizzle of olive or rapeseed oil
500g onions, roughly chopped
Sea salt and freshly ground black pepper
4 cloves garlic, finely chopped

5cm piece fresh ginger, peeled and finely sliced
Zest and juice of 1 orange
400g pre-soaked black beans
1.1 litres hot vegetable stock
1½ heads of broccoli, cut into small florets
Organic short-grain brown rice, to serve

- Preheat the oven to 200°C/400°F/Gas Mark 6. Put the ribs in a roasting tin, put in the oven and roast for about 40 minutes or until they brown, turning them halfway through. Remove and put to one side. Turn the oven down to 170°C/350°F/Gas Mark 4.

- Heat the olive oil in a large lidded ovenproof casserole pot, add the onions and season with the sea salt and freshly ground black pepper. Cook for 4–5 minutes until softened, add the garlic and ginger and cook for a few more minutes, then stir in the orange zest and juice and the soaked black beans. Put the short ribs in the pot along with the stock, and bring to a bubble. Then put the lid on and cook in the oven for 2½ hours, checking on it occasionally and topping up with hot water from the kettle if needed. Remove from the oven and put to one side, and leave it to cool completely.

- Once cold, skim away the layer of fat from the pot – you can use a ladle for this – then take out the ribs, strip the meat from the bones and remove and discard any excess fat. Return the meat and bones to the pot and top up with hot water (about 300ml). Put the lid on and cook for about 1 hour, adding the broccoli and more hot water for the last 30 minutes.

- Remove from the oven, take out the bones, taste, and adjust the seasoning as needed. Serve with the brown rice.

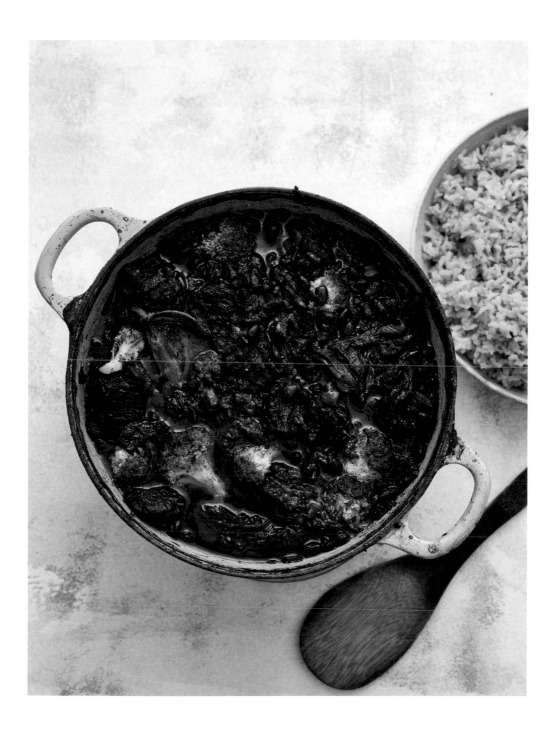

Tarka Dal

If lentils don't make you too gassy (and you'll certainly know if they do!), then this simple veggie dish will keep you feeling full. It's packed with healing spices and I love to scoop it up from the bowl with toasted slices of sourdough. You can get mung dal at most Asian supermarkets but red lentils would work just as well here.

V   SERVES 4–6   428–285 calories

500g mung dal (skinned yellow split mung beans), rinsed in two changes of water
Sea salt and freshly ground black pepper
1 tbsp extra virgin olive oil
1 onion, finely chopped
3 cloves garlic, finely chopped
2 tsp turmeric

Pinch ground cinnamon
Pinch ground cumin
Pinch chilli powder (optional)
400g can chopped tomatoes
Handful of coriander, leaves only
Steamed spinach, to serve

- Put the mung dal in a large pot (the dal will absorb a lot of water and swell, so do use a large one) – a large wide shallow heavy-based pan is good. Add filtered water to cover by half again and bring to the boil, then reduce to a simmer and cook for 30 minutes. Top up with water from the kettle as needed (keep an eye on it – it will need topping up frequently). Skim away any scum from the top as it cooks, and discard. It should be the consistency of soup and nice and creamy. Season well with salt, to taste. You can serve the dal at this stage and just stir in the turmeric, or you can continue the recipe to add the 'tarka' part – either way is tasty.

- While the mung dal is cooking, heat the oil in a large frying pan, add the onion and cook for 3–4 minutes until softened, then stir in the garlic and cook for a few seconds. Now add the turmeric, cinnamon, cumin and chilli (if using) and stir to combine. Season with salt, then tip in the tomatoes and bring to the boil. Simmer for about 10–15 minutes, then add to the pot of dal and stir well to combine. Taste, and season some more if needed.

- Sit the coriander leaves on top, then stir them in when ready to serve. Serve on a bed of steamed spinach.

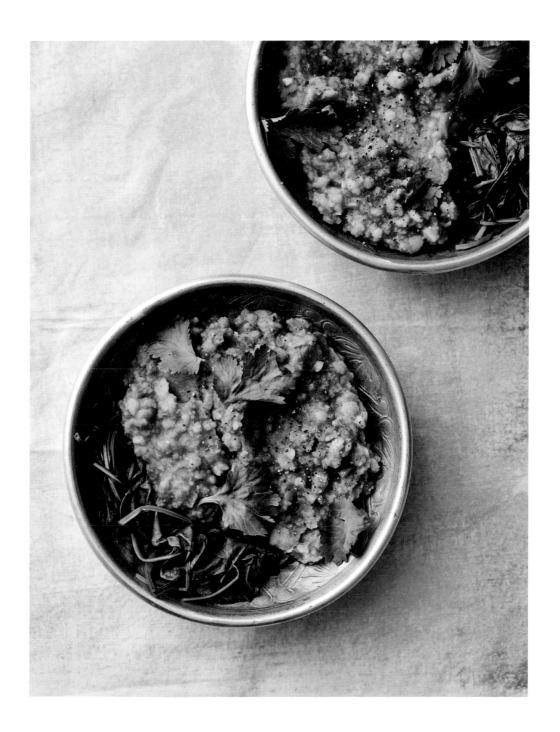

Salmon and Leek Chowder

Tuck into this tasty fish chowder on cooler days – the butter will help soothe your tummy as will the collagen-rich stock. I make a big batch and leave some for the next day, as the flavours intensify and improve the longer you leave it.

SERVES 4   405 calories

½ tbsp extra virgin olive oil

20g organic butter

1 onion, finely chopped

Sea salt and freshly ground black pepper

2 cloves garlic, finely chopped

1 bay leaf

2 leeks (about 200g), trimmed and sliced

A few stalks thyme, leaves only

600g organic potatoes, peeled and cubed

400ml hot fresh fish stock (see page 192)

2 tbsp soured cream

400g wild salmon, skinned

A few parsley stalks, leaves only, finely chopped (optional)

- Heat the oil and butter in a large lidded pan, add the onion and season with the sea salt and freshly ground black pepper. Cook for 3–4 minutes until the onion softens, stir in the garlic and bay leaf and cook for a few seconds more, then add the leeks and the thyme and stir so they absorb all the buttery juices. Cook for 3–4 minutes, then stir in the potatoes.

- Pour in the stock and soured cream and simmer on low with the lid on for about 15 minutes or until the potatoes are tender – top up with a little more hot water if needed.

- Put the fish in whole, continue cooking with the lid on for a further 8 minutes, then take out the fish and flake it into the pan in chunky pieces, stirring gently to combine. To serve, ladle into bowls and sprinkle with the parsley (if using).

LIZ'S TIP

Wild salmon is pricey, but this dish will work well with any firm-fleshed fish. Look for the Marine Stewardship Council (MSC) label for the most sustainable options.

Oxtail Stew

This stew is a veritable feast of gut-healing goodness. Not only do we benefit from all the ingredients, as nothing is poured or boiled away, but they take care of the cooking themselves, leaving us with more downtime to relax and take a break from the kitchen.

 SERVES 4   683 calories

About 2kg oxtail (order from your butcher or farm shop)

Sea salt and freshly ground black pepper

1 tbsp olive or rapeseed oil

1 onion, finely chopped

3 stalks celery, finely chopped

3 star anise

A few rosemary stalks, finely chopped

400g sweet potatoes, peeled and roughly chopped

1 tbsp tamari (gluten-free soy sauce)

900ml hot vegetable stock

½ dark-green cabbage, such as Savoy, shredded

- Preheat the oven to 200°C/400°F/Gas Mark 6. Put the oxtail in a roasting tin, season with the sea salt and freshly ground black pepper, then put in the oven to roast for about 30 minutes or until just turning pale golden. Remove from the oven and put to one side. Turn the heat down to 190°C/375°F/Gas Mark 5.

- Heat the oil in a large lidded ovenproof casserole pot – a cast iron one is good for slow cooking. Add the onion, season and cook for 2–3 minutes, then stir in the celery, star anise and rosemary and cook for a further 2–3 minutes. Stir in the sweet potatoes and cook for a couple of minutes, then put in the oxtail, stir, add the tamari and stir again. Add a little of the stock, turn the heat up and let it bubble, then add the remaining stock and bring to the boil. Reduce to a simmer, put the lid on, then put in the oven for 3 hours.

- Top up with hot water as necessary if it's starting to dry out, then add the cabbage for the last 40 minutes of cooking. Remove from the oven and transfer to shallow bowls, to serve.

Kimchi Marinated Steak

We need protein to help soothe our digestive tract, but it's vital to increase the fibre content in our diets too so as to prevent constipation. I love this easy-to-eat steak dish that's also full of prebiotic fibres, thanks to the garlic, onions, pak choi and kimchi.

  SERVES 4

PREP: OVERNIGHT MARINATING   268 calories

About 600g grass-fed sirloin steak, sliced into strips
1 tbsp olive or rapeseed oil
1 onion, roughly chopped
2 cloves garlic, finely sliced
5cm piece fresh ginger, peeled and finely sliced
1 Chinese (nappa) cabbage, or use a pointed green cabbage, shredded
2 pak choi, trimmed and shredded

Tamari, to taste (optional)
Freshly ground black pepper
4 lemon wedges, to serve

For the marinade:
2 tbsp Kimchi, chopped (page 110; make sure you use plenty of the juice)

- Put the beef in a non-metallic bowl, add the marinade and mix together until really well combined. Cover and leave in the fridge for as long as you have, from 20 minutes to overnight.

- When ready to cook, heat the oil in a wok, add the onion and stir-fry on high, moving it around the pan for a couple of minutes, then add the garlic and ginger and cook for a few seconds, making sure nothing burns.

- Drain the beef strips from the marinade (keeping the marinade to one side), put the beef in the wok and, moving it around the pan, cook on high for a few minutes, then remove it with a slotted spoon and put to one side.

- Put the marinade in the wok, cook for a minute until it bubbles, then add all the greens and continue cooking and stirring until the leaves begin to wilt. Return the beef to the wok and combine everything so it all gets well coated. Taste, and add tamari if it needs it, and some grinds of black pepper.

- Give it a stir, then transfer to serving bowls. Serve with the lemon wedge on the side.

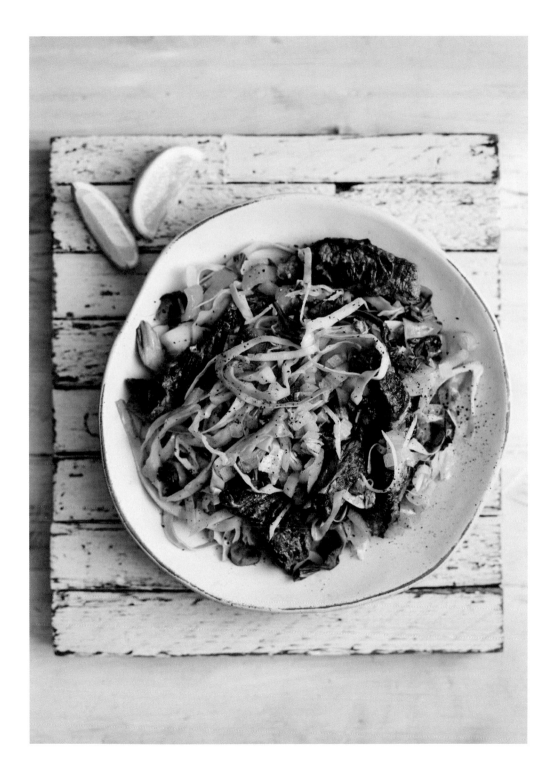

DESSERTS AND TREATS

Blackberry Frozen Yoghurt

This is a fabulously refreshing, fruity dessert. Frozen blackberries are available all year round in the supermarket so you needn't wait until autumn to make this refined-sugar-free frozen yoghurt. And it's a great way to use up your stash of frozen hedgerow-picked berries too.

V GF SERVES 4   193 calories

150g blackberries   1 tbsp water
1 tbsp raw honey   500g plain live Greek yoghurt

- Put the blackberries, honey and water into a pan and heat gently for about 5–6 minutes or until the blackberries begin to split. Remove from the heat and put to one side to cool.

- Put the yoghurt in a food processor and tip in the cooled blackberry mixture, whizz until blended, then spoon out into a shallow container. Put in the freezer and leave for a couple of hours, then remove and scoop it out and put it back into the food processor and whizz again. Return it to the container, cover and put back in the freezer. Once frozen, do this one more time, then cover and leave in the freezer. For the optimum flavour, best eaten within a few weeks.

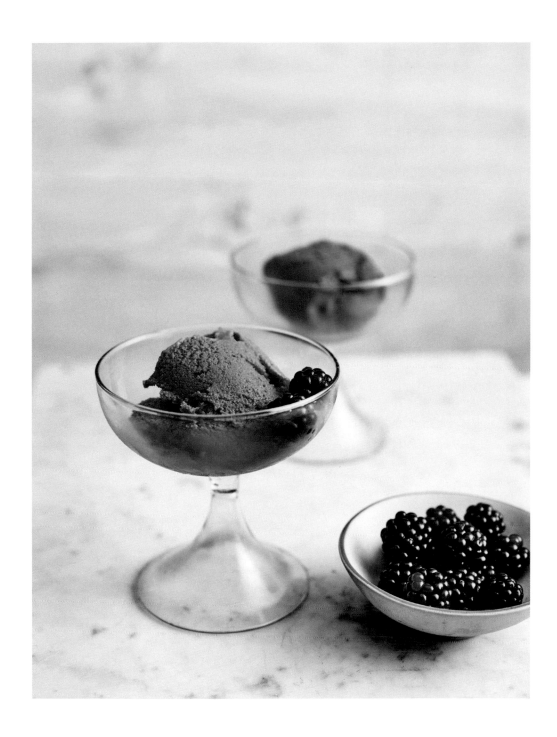

Griddled Pineapple with Ginger and Star Anise

I absolutely love this simple, healthily sweet treat. Pineapple contains the digestion-improving enzyme bromelain, combined here with prebiotic honey and probiotic live yoghurt, plus the spice star anise, which has been used since Roman times as a digestive aid to help minimise stomach upset. Plus it's such a delicious flavour combination – the perfect summer pudding.

 V GF SERVES 4   123 calories

1 ball of stem ginger, finely sliced (reserve a little
   of the syrup)
2 star anise
Juice of 1 orange

½ tsp raw honey
1 fresh pineapple, trimmed, outer skin removed
   and flesh sliced into thin rounds
2 tbsp plain live Greek yoghurt, to serve

- Put the stem ginger and syrup, the star anise, orange juice and honey into a bowl. Add the pineapple and leave for 10 minutes.

- Heat a griddle pan to hot, put in the pineapple slices a few at a time and cook until the underside begins to turn golden and starts to char, then turn and cook the other side. Spoon a little of the juice over it as it cooks. Remove and put to one side and continue to cook all the remaining slices.

- Transfer the pineapple slices to serving plates, remove the star anise from the orange juice mixture and use to decorate, pour over any remaining juice and the ginger slices and serve with a generous dollop of the Greek yoghurt.

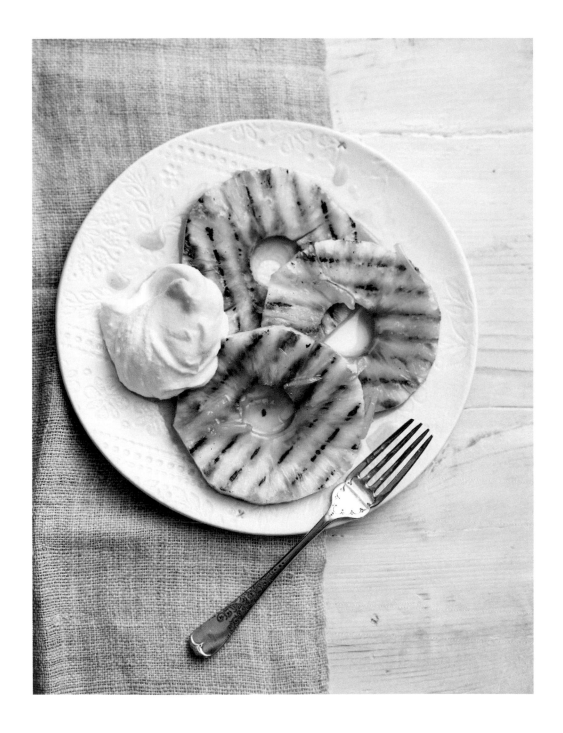

Dark Chocolate and Cardamom Mousse

Who can resist a deliciously fluffy chocolate mousse, especially when it's made with genuine chocolate? This will satisfy every chocolate craving. Even though very dark chocolate does contain sugar, the higher the cocoa percentage, generally the lower the amount of sugar there is. I've used 85 per cent cocoa solids here, and I wouldn't go lower than 70 per cent.

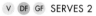 SERVES 2   248 calories

2 organic eggs, separated
60g plain chocolate (85% cocoa), broken into
   pieces
6 cardamom pods, seeds only, crushed
1–2 tsp raw honey (optional)

- Put the egg whites in the bowl of a food mixer, and whisk until fluffy and the mixture has reached soft peaks. Remove and put to one side.

- Put the chocolate and the cardamom in a heatproof bowl, sit it over a pan of simmering water and stir occasionally until it melts.

- With a balloon whisk, whisk the egg yolks into the melted chocolate, then fold in the fluffy egg whites. Taste, and if you need to sweeten, stir in the honey. When all is combined, divide the mixture between two serving dishes and put in the fridge to set and chill for a couple of hours.

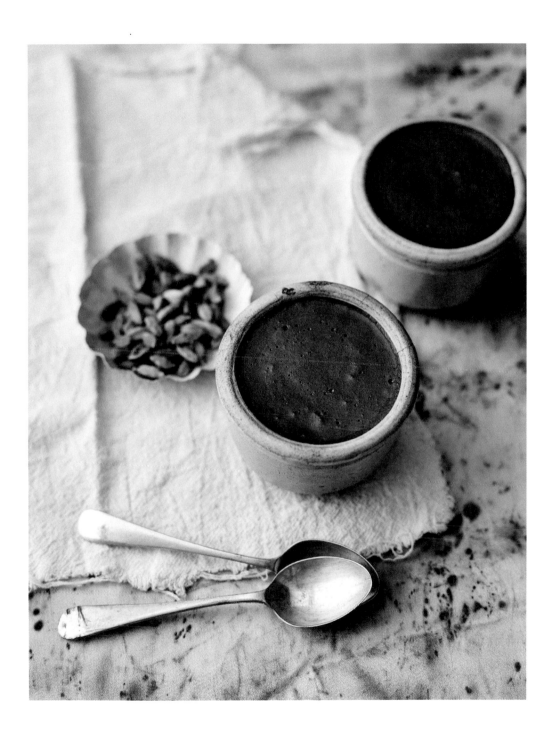

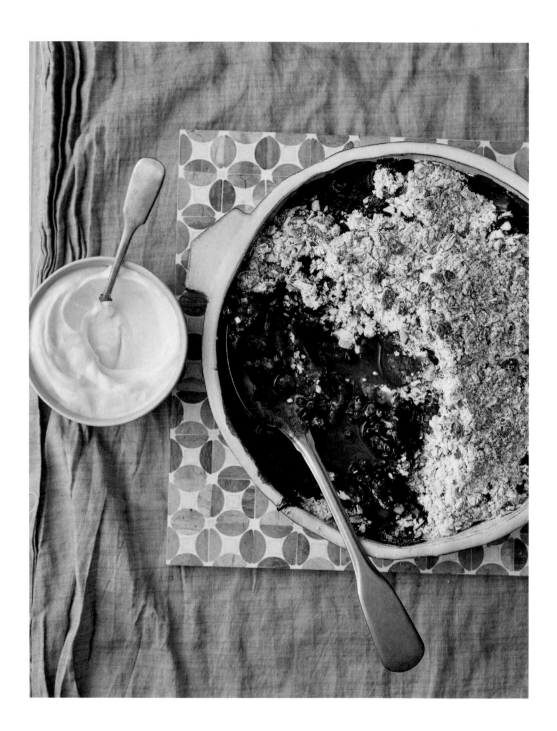

Mixed Berry Gluten-free Crumble

It's so satisfying to make your own crumble – so easy and far healthier than packet versions which are often filled with hydrogenated fats and refined sugars. My gluten-free version is packed to the hilt with zinc and Omega-3-filled seeds (soak them overnight to boost enzyme activity), crunchy nuts and blood-sugar-balancing cinnamon. Enjoy served with a dollop of plain live yoghurt or a drizzle of milk kefir.

V GF SERVES 4–6

PREP: OVERNIGHT SOAKING   496–744 calories

500g fresh or frozen (defrosted) mixed berries:
  e.g. raspberries, blackberries, strawberries,
  redcurrants – add a drizzle of honey or tbsp
  jaggery (raw sugar) if the fruit is really tart
Plain live yoghurt, Milk Kefir (page 106) or crème
  fraîche, to serve

For the crumble topping:
100g flaked almonds, lightly toasted
50g ground almonds
Pinch ground ginger
Pinch cinnamon
100g gluten-free oats (or you can use regular
  porridge oats)
30g pumpkin seeds
30g sunflower seeds
100g rice flour
100g grass-fed butter
1 tbsp muscovado sugar or jaggery

- Preheat the oven to 190°C/375°F/Gas Mark 5. Tip the fruit into a large shallow ovenproof dish and set aside. Drizzle with raw honey or sprinkle with jaggery if the fruit tastes sharp.

- Now make the crumble topping. Put all the ingredients into a food processor and blitz on the pulse setting until mixed, but don't over-mix – you still need some lumps.

- Spoon the crumble topping on top of the fruit to cover, and put it in the oven for about 30–40 minutes or until bubbling and golden. Remove from the oven, spoon into serving dishes and serve with plain live yoghurt or milk kefir – or double cream if it's a special occasion.

Lemon and Camomile Posset

This zesty lemon dessert contains gelatine, rich in collagen to heal the digestive tract in cases of leaky gut. And there are so many new health food brands offering pure, unflavoured gelatine these days, making it very easy to find both in stores and online.

GF SERVES 4

PREP: OVERNIGHT SETTING (OPTIONAL)   178 calories

500g plain live Greek yoghurt
Zest and juice of 2 lemons
10g powdered gelatine (or 2 sheets, broken into pieces)

1 camomile teabag, steeped in 250ml hot water for 10 minutes or until well flavoured
1–2 tsp raw honey, or to taste

- Put the yoghurt into a bowl and stir in the lemon zest and juice. Put to one side.

- Put the gelatine in a bowl and add 50ml of cold water, stir and leave to soften. Then pour in the camomile-infused hot water and whisk the mixture with a fork until lump-free. Pour it into the yoghurt mixture and beat well. Taste, and sweeten to taste with the honey.

- Pour the mixture into individual glass dishes and put in the fridge to set for a few hours or overnight.

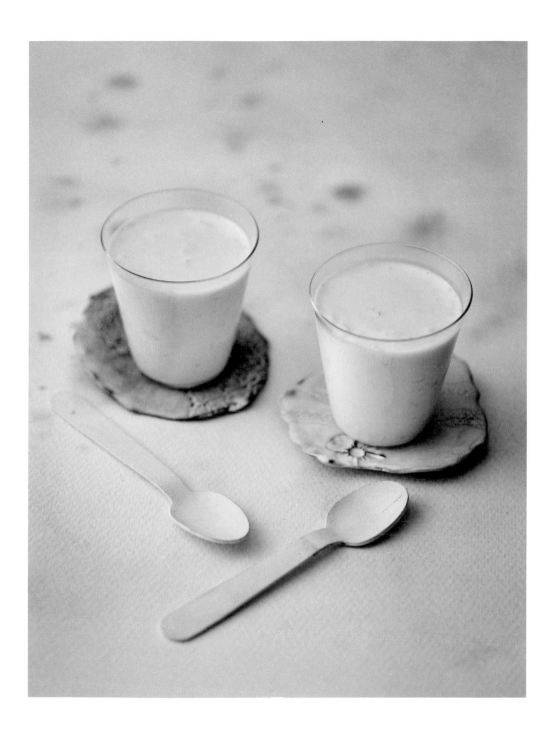

Chocolate Mini-bites

These rich, chocolatey bites will tantalise your tastebuds. The mixture is naturally high in sugar due to the dried fruits as well as the chocolate, so it's a treat best made towards the end of your six-week programme. Also, the addition of avocado and Greek yoghurt boosts the fat content, which will slightly lessen the effects of the sugars. I love to make the slab on a Sunday, then cut it up into small portions to last the family the whole week.

V GF **MAKES 32 MINI-BITES**
PREP: OVERNIGHT SOAKING; OVERNIGHT CHILLING (OPTIONAL)   140 calories

200g plain chocolate (85% cocoa), broken into
   pieces
300g pecan nuts, soaked overnight
150g pitted dates, soaked
150g pitted prunes

For the topping:
100g plain chocolate (85% cocoa)
1 avocado, halved and stoned
1 tbsp plain live Greek yoghurt
1–2 tsp raw honey (optional)

- Put the chocolate pieces into a heatproof bowl, sit it over a pan of simmering water and stir occasionally until melted. Remove and put to one side (keep the bowl and the pan for when you make the topping).

- While the chocolate is melting put the nuts into a food processor and blitz until chopped small, then add the dates and prunes and whizz again. Now add the melted chocolate and mix until really well combined. Spoon into a shallow 30 × 18cm rectangular tin, lined with greaseproof paper overlapping the tin, and flatten until it's even. Put in the fridge to chill while you prepare the topping.

- To make the topping, put the chocolate into the same bowl and sit it over the pan, the water simmering, and heat until melted. Put to one side.

- Put the avocado, yoghurt and honey (if using) into the food processor, then add the melted chocolate and whizz until combined. Spread the mixture over the chocolate and nut slab and put back in the fridge to chill for a few hours or overnight. Lift the slab from the tin using the greaseproof paper and slice into 32 small squares. They will keep in a sealed tin or other container for up to a week.

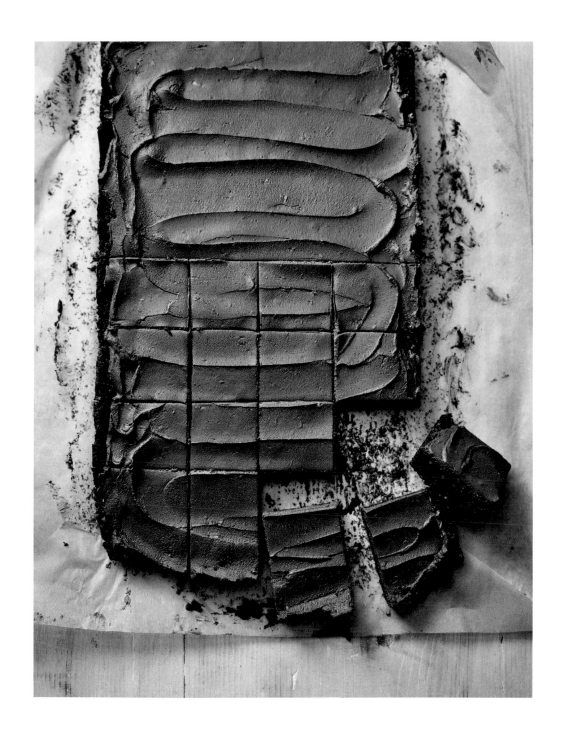

Coconut and Apple Ice Cream

There are a few steps involved in this ice-cream recipe – but trust me, it's worth it! The fruity apple balances so well with the coconut, plus it's another way to make the most of your probiotic-packed homemade kefir.

Ⓥ ⒼⒻ SERVES 4–6   551–367 calories

100g pack coconut chunks
2 eating apples, peeled, cored and roughly
   chopped
250ml double cream

25g coconut sugar
3 organic egg yolks
250ml Milk Kefir (page 106)

- Preheat the oven to 190°C/375°F/Gas Mark 5. Tip the coconut chunks into a roasting tin and put in the oven for 10–15 minutes or until golden brown. Remove and put into a food processor and blitz until well chopped, leaving plenty of texture.

- While the coconut is roasting, put the apples in a pan along with a sprinkle of water, just enough so they don't burn. Heat gently for about 10 minutes until they just begin to soften, then add to the food processor with the coconut and whizz again until blended. Put to one side to cool.

- Put the cream in the pan and heat gently until it just boils, then tip in the sugar and stir for a minute or two until it has dissolved. Remove from the heat and whisk in the egg yolks until the mixture begins to thicken slightly, then pour it through a sieve into a bowl and leave it to cool. Now stir in the milk kefir and the apple and coconut mixture.

- Transfer it to a freezer-proof container – a flat one will allow it to freeze more quickly. Cover and put in the freezer for a couple of hours, then remove and spoon into the food processor and whizz until well mixed. Tip it back into the container, cover, and put back in the freezer. Repeat this once more, and serve once it's frozen.

- Remove from the freezer 5 minutes before serving to allow it to soften slightly. Serve as scoops in cold glass serving dishes.

Labneh with Papaya and Honey

Labneh is a full-fat yoghurt dish that originates from the Middle East. It's different from regular yoghurt in that it's been strained so as to remove the watery whey, leaving a thicker, creamier consistency. It's perfectly complemented by sweeter fruits such as papaya, especially if you also use the seeds, which are good for aiding digestion.

V GF **SERVES 4**
PREP: OVERNIGHT STRAINING   231 calories

500g plain live Greek yoghurt
2 papayas, halved, peeled, deseeded, flesh sliced
4–6 tsp raw honey

- Sit a plastic sieve over a large bowl, then line the sieve with a large piece of muslin cloth. Spoon in the yoghurt, then bring the cloth sides together and tie so that you have a muslin ball. Suspend the ball (or bag) over the bowl and sieve, and leave to strain overnight.

- The yoghurt in the muslin ball should become quite firm, like a cream cheese – this is the labneh (the whey has dripped away into the bowl).

- Divide the labneh up between serving plates, add the sliced papaya and drizzle over the honey, to serve. Any leftover labneh can be kept in the fridge for a couple of days.

LIZ'S TIP

To preserve the labneh and serve it later as a savoury bite, roll into individual balls about the size of a walnut and pop into a clean, sterilised jar. Fill to the brim with olive or rapeseed oil and seal. Store it in the fridge for a couple of days.

Goat's Cheese and Honey Cheesecake Topped with Berries

Cheesecake makes me smile! It's one of those comfort foods guaranteed to hit the spot, especially the baked variety, which always seems fluffier and somehow more satisfying. This refined-sugar-free version is reassuringly simple too, and I know you're going to love it. A delicious celebration cake.

 SERVES 12

PREP: OVERNIGHT CHILLING   *139 calories*

5 organic eggs, separated
300g soft goat's cheese, roughly chopped
Zest and juice of 2 lemons
1 tbsp raw honey (use more if you like it sweeter)
3 tbsp rice flour
Drizzle of double cream or crème fraîche,
   to serve (optional)

For the topping:
About 300g mixed berries, frozen (defrosted) or
   fresh – strawberries, raspberries, blueberries or
   blackberries

- Preheat the oven to 170°C/350°F/Gas Mark 4. Prepare a deep round 20cm loose- or spring-bottomed tin, lightly greased and the base lined with greaseproof paper. Put the egg whites in the bowl of a food mixer and whisk until fluffy and doubled in volume. Spoon out into a clean bowl and put to one side.

- Put the goat's cheese into the mixer bowl, add the lemon zest and juice and the honey and beat using the beaters. Taste to see if sweet enough or lemony enough and adjust as needed. Now add the egg yolks and beat again until well combined. Fold in the egg whites, then fold in the flour.

- Spoon into the prepared tin, level the top and put in the oven to bake for 30 minutes. The top may still be a little wobbly, but don't worry as it will continue to cook. It may also crack – again, don't worry, this often happens with cheesecake.

- Remove from the oven and leave to cool completely, then sit the tin in the fridge overnight to chill. Run a knife around the inside edge of the tin to release the cheesecake and sit it on a serving plate. Spoon over the fruit and slice.

- Serve alone or, if you like, with a drizzle of cream or a dollop of crème fraîche.

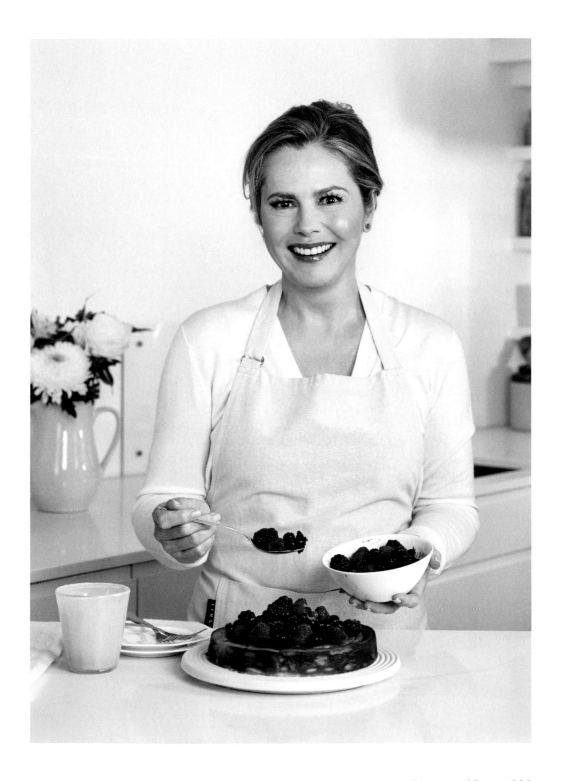

Courgette and Apple Cake

Packed with pecans and prunes as well as apple and courgette, a piece of this cake is possibly one of your five a day! You can make it gluten-free too, if you wish, by replacing the spelt flour with almond flour.

v SERVES 12   311 calories

200g organic butter, softened
180g dark-brown muscovado sugar
2 organic eggs, lightly beaten
200g organic wholegrain spelt flour (mixed with
    1 tsp baking powder)
250g (about 2 large) grated courgette
1 apple, grated
100g prunes, chopped
50g pecan nuts, soaked and chopped

To serve:
Crème fraîche or plain Greek yoghurt (optional)
Apple batons (optional)

Equipment: A 1-litre loaf tin, about 23 × 12 ×
    7cm, lightly greased and the base lined with
    greaseproof paper

- Preheat the oven to 170°C/350°F/Gas Mark 4. Put the butter and sugar into a food mixer and, using the beaters, beat until creamy – about 10 minutes. Add the eggs a little at a time, beating after each addition (add a spoonful of flour to stop it curdling), then beat in half the flour and stir the rest in with a spoon.

- Now stir in the courgette, apple, prunes and pecan nuts and spoon into the prepared tin.

- Put in the oven and bake for 1 hour or until golden and risen and when a skewer poked into it comes out clean. Remove the cake and leave it to cool in the tin for 10 minutes, then loosen the edges and turn out onto a wire rack.

- Leave it to cool, then slice. Serve on its own or, if you like, with a spoonful of crème fraîche or Greek yoghurt and a few crunchy apple batons.

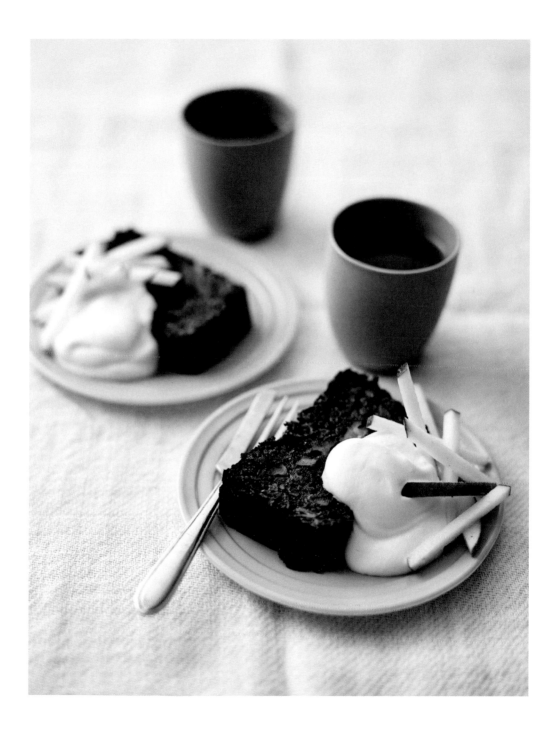

DRINKS

Apple, Berry and Beetroot Juice with Kombucha

I agree, kombucha can be an acquired taste. We've become so used to over-sweet foods that here in the so-called developed world we've lost our appetite for more tangy, unusual flavours. But you can reap all the benefits of kombucha and help your tastebuds adjust by mixing it with energising beetroot juice, berries and apple, as I do here.

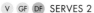 SERVES 2   112 calories

225g blueberries
150g raspberries
2 small (150g) raw beetroots, trimmed
1 apple, roughly chopped
100ml Kombucha (page 104)

Equipment: Juicer machine

- Feed the blueberries into the juicer machine, followed by the raspberries, beetroots and apple, then mix the juices together. Add the kombucha to the juice and mix again. Transfer to a jug and put in the fridge to chill before serving.

LIZ'S TIP

All the juice recipes in this book are tested using a juicer which separates the juice from the fibre so you end up with just the juice. If you're using a blender-style juicer the drink will be of a thicker consistency, but just as delicious.

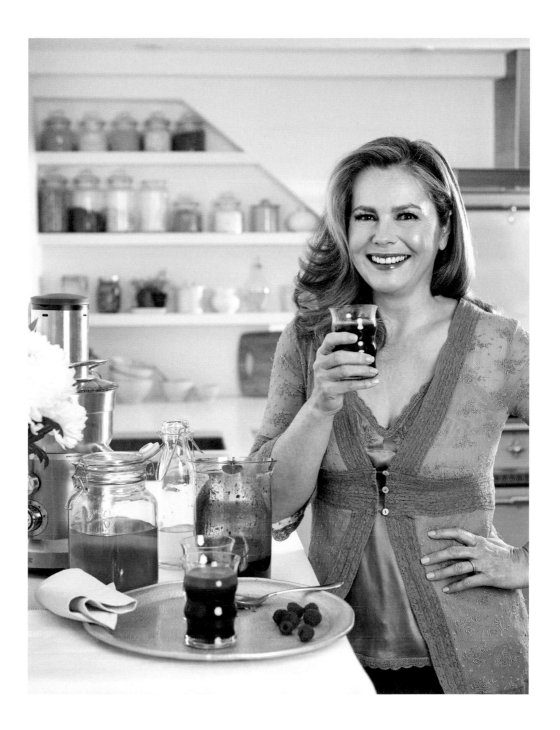

Banana, Prune and Almond Smoothie

This will get your gut working – no question! Bananas are packed with prebiotic fibre and prunes are of course renowned for helping to 'keep things regular'.

Ⓥ ⒼⒻ MAKES 500ML   290 calories

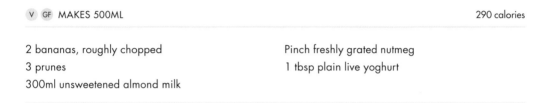

2 bananas, roughly chopped
3 prunes
300ml unsweetened almond milk

Pinch freshly grated nutmeg
1 tbsp plain live yoghurt

- Put all the ingredients into a high-powered blender and blend on high until well combined. Pour into a jug and put in the fridge to chill before serving.

Homemade Almond Milk with Cinnamon and Honey

I love making my own almond milk, especially as some of the shop-bought versions can contain as little as 2 per cent almonds!

Ⓥ ⒹⒻ ⒼⒻ MAKES ABOUT 500ML
          PREP: OVERNIGHT SOAKING   194 calories

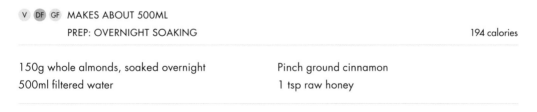

150g whole almonds, soaked overnight
500ml filtered water

Pinch ground cinnamon
1 tsp raw honey

- Strain the almonds and add them to a high-powered blender along with the water. Blend for a minute or so until well mixed, then add the cinnamon and honey and blend for about 5 minutes.
- Sit a large piece of muslin cloth over a sieve placed over a bowl and strain the almond mixture through the cloth. Pour the milk into a jug and put in the fridge to chill before serving.

Green Juice

Green is undoubtedly the colour of health and wellness, which is exactly what you'll get when you drink this cleansing juice. The chlorophyll-packed leaves plus lime juice help to alkalise your gut – try a small cupful each day, sipped slowly first thing, for two weeks while you detox your diet.

 V DF GF **SERVES 2**   194 calories

2 stalks celery, roughly chopped   *Equipment:* Juicer machine
2 apples, roughly chopped
Handful of spinach leaves
150g kale leaves, tough stalks removed
½ lime
2cm piece fresh ginger

• Feed everything into the juicer machine, then mix the juices together. Pour into two serving glasses and put in the fridge to chill before serving.

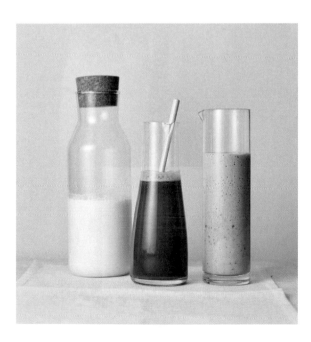

Turmeric, Lime and Honey Tea

Turmeric truly is a wonder spice – anti-inflammatory and rejuvenating – and what better way to soak up all the healing benefits than with the raw grated root? This cleansing and antioxidant-packed tea may well become your new brew of choice! Use powdered turmeric if you can't find the fresh root.

V DF GF **SERVES 1**   12 calories

8g fresh turmeric root, peeled and finely grated using a microplane (wear food gloves or rubber gloves to do this, as turmeric will stain your nails)

400ml hot filtered water (not boiling)
Juice of ½ lime or lemon
1 tsp raw honey

Put the turmeric into a mug, pour in the hot water and stir well, then squeeze in the lime or lemon juice and stir in the honey. Sip while warm – and do drink up all the bits of turmeric.

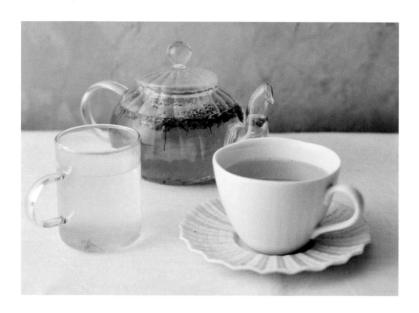

Fennel and Ginger Tea

There are so many good tea blends that can soothe and calm the gut, particularly camomile and fennel, which is why I've included those here as some of my favourites.

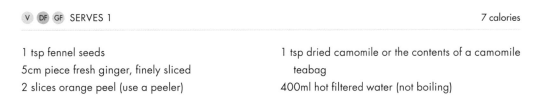

V DF GF SERVES 1   7 calories

1 tsp fennel seeds
5cm piece fresh ginger, finely sliced
2 slices orange peel (use a peeler)

1 tsp dried camomile or the contents of a camomile teabag
400ml hot filtered water (not boiling)

- Add everything to a small teapot and pour over the water. Leave to steep for 5 minutes, then pour through a strainer to serve.

Camomile and Lavender Tea

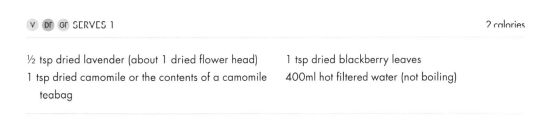

V DF GF SERVES 1   2 calories

½ tsp dried lavender (about 1 dried flower head)
1 tsp dried camomile or the contents of a camomile teabag

1 tsp dried blackberry leaves
400ml hot filtered water (not boiling)

- Put the lavender, camomile and blackberry leaves into a small teapot and pour over the hot water. Leave to steep for 5 minutes, then strain, to serve.

Fresh Herb and Fruit Teas

With just a few windowbox herbs and a bowlful of citrus fruits, you can concoct a variety of healing teas such as these . . .

Rosemary and Lemon

V DF GF SERVES 2   7 calories

A few stalks fresh rosemary, leaves finely chopped
2 pieces lemon peel (use a peeler)
400ml hot filtered water (not boiling)

- Put the rosemary and lemon into a small teapot. Pour over the water and leave to steep for 5 minutes, then strain, to serve.

Sage and Orange

V DF GF SERVES 2   2 calories

About 3–4 fresh sage leaves, roughly torn
2 pieces orange peel (use a peeler)
400ml hot filtered water (not boiling)

- Put the sage and orange into a small teapot. Pour over the water and leave to steep for 5 minutes, then strain, to serve.

Mint and Lime

V DF GF SERVES 2   7 calories

Handful of fresh mint leaves
1 piece lime peel (use a peeler)
400ml hot filtered water (not boiling)

- Put the mint and lime into a small teapot. Pour over the water and leave to steep for 5 minutes, then strain, to serve.

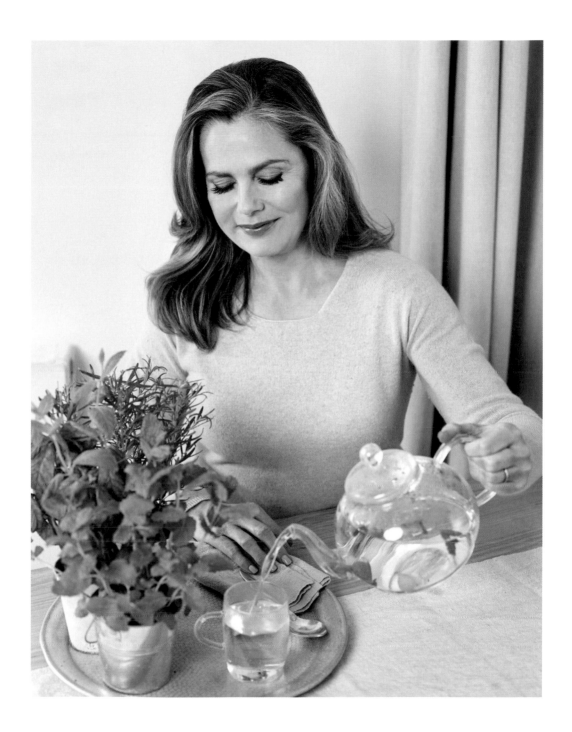

Raspberry Kvass with Honey

Such an easy drink to make, kvass is fast becoming the popular fermented beverage *du jour* – this raspberry version is absolutely perfect served over ice on a summer's day.

 V DF GF MAKES 1 LITRE
PREP: FERMENTING TIME (2–3 DAYS)   11 calories

200g organic or homegrown raspberries
2 tsp raw honey
About 700ml filtered water

Equipment: A 1-litre sterilised sealable jar

- Put the raspberries and honey into the jar, pour in the water, leaving a little room at the top. Seal and leave for 2–3 days, giving it a shake a few times a day. It should start to bubble, which means it has started to ferment. Have a taste – it should be sweet and tangy. Strain into a jug and put into the fridge to chill before serving. It will keep in the fridge for up to 1 week.

Mango and Coconut Lassi

Lassi is popular in Indian cuisine. This refined-sugar-free version provides a healthy dose of probiotics and you could even use Milk Kefir (page 106) instead of the plain coconut milk.

V GF MAKES 900ML   409 calories

2 ice cubes
4 cardamom pods, seeds only
Pinch freshly ground black pepper
100ml unsweetened coconut milk drink (from
  a carton)

100ml buttermilk
2 tbsp plain live yoghurt
500g fresh mango, roughly chopped

- Put the ice into a high-powered blender along with the cardamom and black pepper and blitz until crushed, then add the coconut milk, buttermilk, yoghurt and mango and blend well until all combined. Pour into a jug and put in the fridge to chill before serving.

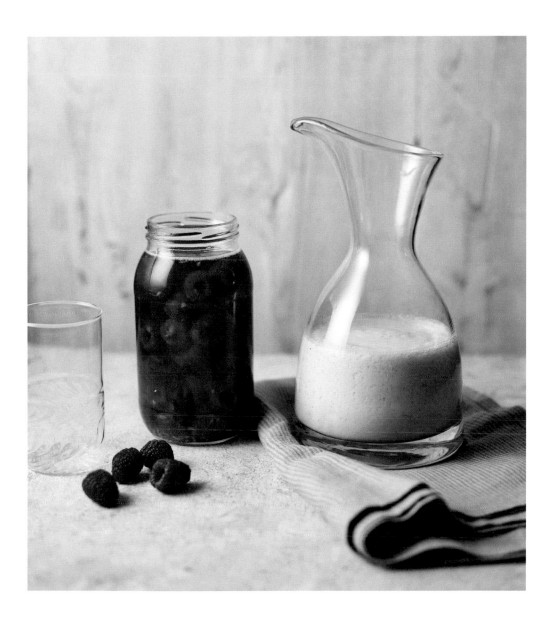

Stomach-soothing Shots

Once you've tasted these, you may never want an alcoholic shot again . . . Use your juicer machine to make drinks that will flood your body with so much goodness. Chin-chin!

Carrot and Fennel

V DF GF SERVES 4   20 calories

Small fennel bulb (150g), trimmed and roughly
   chopped
400g carrots, peeled and roughly chopped
1 orange, peel and pith removed, roughly
   chopped

- Feed the fennel into the juicer machine, add
  the carrots and then the orange. Mix well,
  then pour into a small jug or shot glasses
  and put in the fridge to chill before serving.

Spinach and Pineapple

V DF GF SERVES 4   40 calories

100g spinach
1 piece fresh turmeric, peeled
1 fresh pineapple, trimmed and skinned, roughly
   chopped

- Put the spinach into the feeder of the
  juicer machine, then add the turmeric and
  pineapple. Mix well, then pour into a small
  jug or shot glasses and put in the fridge to
  chill before serving.

Pink Grapefruit and Ginger

V DF GF SERVES 2   20 calories

1 pink grapefruit, peel and pith removed, roughly
   chopped
2.5cm piece fresh ginger, peeled and roughly
   chopped
½ tsp raw honey (optional)

- Feed the grapefruit into the juicer, and then
  the ginger. Mix well and taste – stir through
  the honey if you really need the sweetness.
  Pour into shot glasses and chill in the fridge
  before serving.

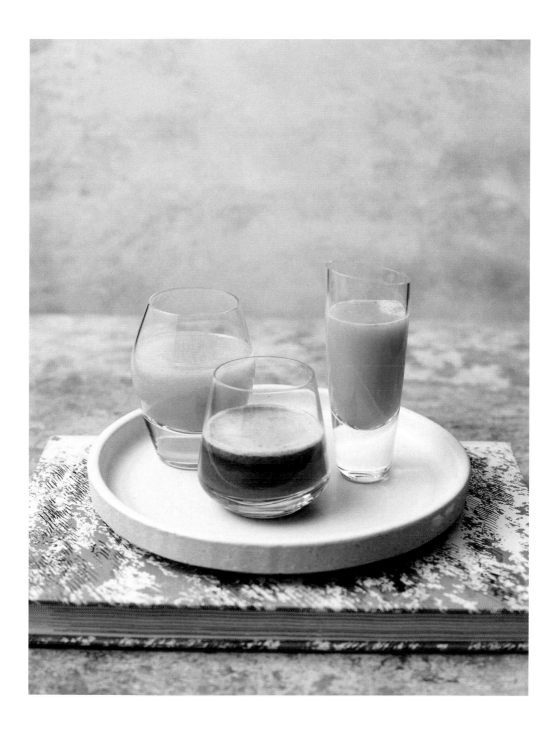

Notes

INTRODUCTION

p. 10   http://britishgut.org Canny, G. O. & McCormick, B. A., 'Bacteria in the Intestine, a Helpful Resident or an Enemy from Within?, *Infection and Immunity*, 78/6 (2008), 3360–73

p. 12   Inman, M., 'How Bacteria Turn Fiber into Food', *PLoS Biology*, 9/12 (2011)

p. 12   Bollinger, R. R. et al., 'Biofilms in the Large Bowel Suggest an Apparent Function of the Human Vermiform Appendix', *Journal of Theoretical Biology*, 249/4 (2007), 826–31

p. 13   http://www.londonhealth.co.uk/digestive/irritable-bowel-syndrome-ibs.html

p. 15   Collen, A., *10% Human: How Your Body's Microbes Hold the Key to Health and Happiness* (New York, 2015)

p. 15   http://medicalxpress.com/news/2016-10-links-protein-wheat-inflammation-chronic.html

p. 16   www.who.int/gho/ncd/risk_factors/overweight/en

p. 16   Speliotes, E. K. et al., 'Association Analyses of 249, 796 Individuals Reveal 18 New Loci Associated with Body Mass Index', *Nature Genetics*, 42/11 (2010), 937–48

p. 16   Weston, D., *Infection Prevention and Control: Theory and Clinical Practice for Healthcare Professionals* (Chichester, England, 2008)

p. 16   Goodrich, Julia K., et al, 'Human Genetics Shape the Gut Microbiome' 159 (4), (2014), 789–799

p. 19   http://textbookofbacteriology.net/normalflora.html

p. 19   Cogen, A. L., Nizet, V. & Gallo, R. L., 'Skin Microbiota: A Source of Disease or Defence?', *The British Journal of Dermatology*, 158/3 (2008), 442–55

WEEK ONE

p. 23   Jabr, F., 'The Food Fight in Your Gut; Why Bacteria Will Change the Way You Think about Calories', *Scientific American* (12 September 2012) <https://blogs.scientificamerican.com/brainwaves/the-food-fight-in-your-guts-why-bacteria-will-change-the-way-you-think-about-calories/>

p. 24   Suez, J. et al., 'Artificial Sweeteners Induce Glucose Intolerance by Altering the Gut Microbiota', *Nature*, 514/7521 (2014), 181–6

p. 24   Krüger, M. et al., 'Glysophate Suppresses the Antagonistic Effect of Enterococcus Spp. on Clostridium Botulinum', *Anaerobe*, 20 (2013), 74–8

p. 24   Shehata, A. A. et al., 'The Effect of Glysophate on Potential Pathogens and Beneficial Members of Poultry Microbiota in Vitro', *Current Microbiology*, 66/4 (2012), 350–8

p. 24   Guarner, F. & Malagelada, J. R., 'Gut Flora in Health and Disease', *Lancet*, 361/9356 (2003), 512–9

p. 24   Samsel, A. & Seneff, S., 'Glyphosate's Suppression of Cytochrome P450 Enzymes and Amino Acid Biosynthesis by the Gut Microbiome: Pathways to Modern Diseases', *Entropy*, 15/4 (2013), 1416–63

p. 24   Williams, G. M., Kroes, R. & Munro, I. C., 'Safety Evaluation and Risk Assessment of the Herbicide Roundup and Its Active Ingredient, Glyphosate, for Humans', *Regulatory Toxicology and Pharmacology*, 31/2 (2000), 117–65

p. 24   Samsel, A. & Seneff, S., 'Glyphosate, Pathways to Modern Diseases II: Celiac Sprue and Gluten Intolerance', *Interdisciplinary Toxicology*, 6/4 (2014), 159–84

p. 26   Haydel, S. E., Remenih, C. M. & Williams, L. B., 'Broad-Spectrum in Vitro Antibacterial Activities of Clay Minerals against Antibiotic-Susceptible and Antibiotic-Resistant Bacterial Pathogens', *The Journal of Antimicrobial Chemotherapy*, 61/2 (2007), 353–61

p. 29   Sienkiewicz, M., Wasiela, M. & Głowacka, A., 'The Antibacterial Activity of Oregano Essential Oil (Origanum Heracleoticum L.) against Clinical Strains of Escherichia Coli and Pseudomonas Aeruginosa', *Medycyna Doswiadczalna I Mikrobiologia*, 64/4 (2012), 297–307

p. 30   http://universityhealthnews.com/daily/nutrition/grapefruit-seed-extract-uses-and-benefits

p. 30   Markin, D., Duek, L. & Berdicevsky, I., 'In Vitro Antimicrobial Activity of Olive Leaves', *Mycoses*, 46/3–4 (2003), 132–6

p. 32   Ranasinghe, P. et al., 'Medicinal Properties of "True" Cinnamon (Cinnamomum Zeylanicum): A Systematic Review', *BMC Complementary and Alternative Medicine*, 13 (2013) 275

WEEK TWO

p. 37   'Boost C-Section Babies by Giving Them Vaginal Bacteria', *New Scientist* (1 February 2016) <https://www.newscientist.com/article/2075768-boost-c-section-babies-by-giving-them-vaginal-bacteria/>

p. 38   Pearce, M. et al., 'Changes in objectively measured BMI in children aged 4–11 years: Data from the National Child Measurement Programme,' *Journal of Public Health* (2015).

p. 38   Davies, M., 'Children Given Antibiotics Before the Age of Two "Are More Likely to Be Obese by Five", *Mail Online* (3 October 2014) <www.dailymail.co.uk/health/article-2779251/Children-given-antibiotics-age-two-likely-obese-five.html>

p. 39   McVey Neufeld, K. A. et al., 'Reframing the Teenage Wasteland: Adolescent Microbiota–Gut–Brain Axis', *Canadian Journal of Psychiatry*, 61/4 (2016), 214–21

p. 39   Fisher, L., '6 Weird Effects Fast Food Has on Your Brain', *Reader's Digest* (30 June 2014) <http://www.rd.com/health/wellness/effects-of-fast-food/>

p. 40   Kort, R. et al., 'Shaping the Oral Microbiota through Intimate Kissing', *Microbiome*, 2/1 (2014), 41

p. 41   Mulak, A., Taché, Y. & Larauche, M., 'Sex Hormones in the Modulation of Irritable Bowel Syndrome', *World Journal of Gastroenterology*, 20/10 (2014), 2433–48

p. 41   Parma, M. et al., ''The Role of Vaginal Lactobacillus Rhamnosus (Normogin®) in Preventing Bacterial Vaginosis in Women with History of Recurrences, Undergoing Surgical Menopause: A Prospective Pilot Study', *European Review for Medical and Pharmacological Sciences*, 17/10 (2013), 1399–1403

p. 41   Xu, W.L. et al., 'Midlife Overweight and Obesity Increase Late-Life Dementia Risk', *Neurology*, 76/18 (2011), 1568–74

p. 41   Distrutti, E. et al., 'Modulation of Intestinal Microbiota by the Probiotic VSL#3 Resets Brain Gene Expression and Ameliorates the Age-Related Deficit in LTP', *PLoS One*, 9/9 (2014)

p. 41   Pérez Martínez, G., Bäuerl, C. & Collado, M. C., 'Understanding Gut Microbiota in Elderly's Health Will Enable Intervention through Probiotics', *Beneficial Microbes*, 5/3 (2014), 235–46

p. 41   'Parkinson's May Begin in Gut and Spread to the Brain Via the Vagus Nerve', *Neuroscience News* (23 June 2015) <http://neurosciencenews.com/parkinsons-gastrointestinal-tract-neurology-2150/>

p. 42   Fiala, M. et al., '3 Supplementation Increases Amyloid Phagocytosis and Resolvin D1 in Patients with Minor Cognitive Impairment', *FASEB Journal*, 29/7 (2015), 2681–9

p. 47   de la Monte, S. M. & Wands, J. R., 'Alzheimer's Disease Is Type 3 Diabetes—Evidence Reviewed', *Journal of Diabetes Science and Technology*, 2/6 (2008), 1101–13

p. 48   Scheibye-Knudsen, M. et al., 'A High-Fat Diet and NAD(+) Activate Sirt1 to Rescue Premature Aging in Cockayne Syndrome', *Cell Metabolism*, 20/5 (2014), 840–55

p. 48   Korting, H. C. & Braun-Falco, O., 'The Effect of Detergents on Skin pH and Its Consequences', *Clinics in Dermatology* 14/1 (1996) 23–7

p. 48   Sinclair Drake, K. & Finch, H.G., 'Mild Acidity Promotes Healthy Skin Microflora and Dermal Longevity,' (2016). Scribd.com

WEEK THREE

p. 52   Langdon, A., Crook, N. & Dantas, G., 'The Effects of Antibiotics on the Microbiome throughout Development and Alternative Approaches for Therapeutic Modulation', *Genome Medicine*, 8 (2016), 39

p. 52   Sanders, M. E. & Klaenhammer, T. R., 'Invited Review: The Scientific Basis of Lactobacillus Acidophilus NCFM Functionality as a Probiotic', *Journal of Dairy Science*, 84/2 (2001), 319–31

p. 52   Gibson, G. R., McCartney, A. L. & Rastall, R. A., 'Prebiotics and Resistance to Gastrointestinal Infections', *British Journal of Nutrition*, 93/S1 (2005), S31–4

p. 52   Nobaek, S. et al., 'Alteration of Intestinal Microflora Is Associated with Reduction in Abdominal Bloating and Pain in Patients with Irritable Bowel Syndrome', *The American Journal of Gastroenterology*, 95/5 (2000), 1231–38

p. 52   Walker, W. A., 'Role of Nutrients and Bacterial Colonization in the Development of Intestinal Host Defense', *Journal of Pediatric Gastroenterology and Nutrition*, 30/S2 (2000), S2–7

p. 52   Vanderhoof, J. A., 'Probiotics and Intestinal Inflammatory Disorders in Infants and Children', *Journal of Pediatric Gastroenterology and Nutrition*, 30/S2 (2000), S34–8

p. 52   Schultz, M. & Sartor, R. B., 'Probiotics and Inflammatory Bowel Diseases', *American Journal of Gastroenterology*, 95/S1 (2000), S19–21

p. 52   Marteau, P. R. et al., 'Protection from Gastrointestinal Diseases with the Use of Probiotics', *American Journal of Clinical Nutrition*, 73/S2 (2001), S430–436 and Shornikova, A. V. et al., 'Lactobacillus Reuteri as a Therapeutic Agent in Acute Diarrhea in Young Children', *Journal of Pediatric Gastroenterology and Nutrition*, 24/4 (1997), 399–404

p. 52   Martinez, R. C. et al., 'Improved Treatment of Vulvovaginal Candidiasis with Fluconazole plus Probiotic Lactobacillus Rhamnosus GR-1 and Lactobacillus Reuteri RC-14', *Letters in Applied Microbiology*, 48/3 (2009), 269–74

p. 52   Anukam, K. et al., 'Augmentation of Antimicrobial Metronidazole Therapy of Bacterial Vaginosis with Oral Probiotic Lactobacillus Rhamnosus GR-1 and Lactobacillus Reuteri RC-14: Randomized, Double-Blind, Placebo Controlled Trial', *Microbes and Infection*, 8/6 (2006), 1450–4

p. 52   http://www.exploresupplements.com/understanding-probiotics-basics-type

p. 52   Manley, K. J. et al., 'Probiotic Treatment of Vancomycin-Resistant Enterococci: A Randomised Controlled Trial', *The Medical Journal of Australia*, 186/9 (2007), 454–7

p. 52   Tomioka, H., Sato, K. & Saito, H., 'The Protective Activity of Immunostimulants against Listeria Monocytogenes Infection in Mice', *Journal of Medical Microbiology*, 36/2 (1992), 112–6

p. 52   Bravo, J. A. et al., 'Ingestion of Lactobacillus Strain Regulates Emotional Behavior and Central GABA Receptor Expression in a Mouse via the Vagus Nerve', *Proceedings of the National Academy of Sciences USA*, 108/38 (2011) 16050–5

p. 52   Marteau, P. R. et al., 'Protection from Gastrointestinal Diseases with the Use of Probiotics', *American Journal of Clinical Nutrition*, 73/S2 (2001), S430–6

p. 53   Waitzberg, D. L. et al., 'The Effect of Probiotic Fermented Milk that Includes Bifidobacterium Lactis CNCM I-2494 on the Reduction of Gastrointestinal Discomfort and Symptoms in Adults: A Narrative Review', *Nutrición Hospitalaria*, 32/2 (2015), 501–9

p. 53   Chenoll, E. B. et al., 'Novel Probiotic Bifidobacterium Bifidum CECT 7366 Strain Active against the Pathogenic Bacterium Helicobacter Pylori', *Applied and Environmental Microbiology*, 77/4 (2010), 1335–43

p. 53   Langhendries, J. P. et al., 'Effect of a Fermented Infant Formula Containing Viable Bifidobacteria on the Fecal Flora Composition and pH of Healthy Full-Term Infants', *Journal of Pediatric Gastroenterology and Nutrition*, 21/2 (1995), 177–81

p. 53   Turroni, F. et al., 'Ability of Bifidobacterium Breve to Grow on Different Types of Milk: Exploring the Metabolism of Milk through Genome Analysis', *Applied and Environmental Microbiology*, 77/20 (2011), 7408–17

p. 53   Tabbers, M. M. et al., 'Is Bifidobacterium Breve Effective in the Treatment of Childhood Constipation? Results from a Pilot Study', *Nutrition Journal*, 10/1 (2011), 19

p. 53   www.fda.gov/downloads/Food/IngredientsPackagingLabeling/GRAS/NoticeInventory/UCM346881

p. 53   http://www.exploresupplements.com/understanding-probiotics-basics-type

p. 53   Asahara, T. et al., 'Probiotic Bifidobacteria Protect Mice from Lethal Infection with Shiga Toxin-Producing Escherichia Coli O157: H7', *Infection and Immunity*, 72/4 (2004), 2240–4

p. 53   Taylor, J. R. & Mitchell, D., *The Wonder of Probiotics: A 30-Day Plan to Boost Energy, Enhance Weight Loss, Heal GI Problems, Prevent Disease, and Slow Aging* (New York, 2008)

p. 53   Whitford, E. J. et al., 'Effects of Streptococcus Thermophilus TH-4 on Intestinal Mucositis Induced by the Chemotherapeutic Agent, 5-Fluorouracil (5-FU)', *Cancer Biology & Therapy*, 8/6 (2009), 505–11

p. 53   Everard, A. et al., 'Cross-Talk between Akkermansia Muciniphila and Intestinal Epithelium Controls Diet-Induced Obesity', *Proceedings of the National Academy of Sciences USA*, 110/22 (2013), 9066–71

p. 56   Heap, S. et al., 'Eight-Day Consumption of Inulin Added to a Yogurt Breakfast Lowers Postprandial Appetite Ratings but Not Energy Intakes in Young Healthy Females: A Randomised Controlled Trial', *British Journal of Nutrition*, 115/2 (2016), 262–70

p. 56   Moreno Franco, B. et al., 'Soluble and Insoluble Dietary Fibre Intake and Risk Factors for CVD and Metabolic Syndrome in Middle-Aged Adults: The AWHS Cohort', *Nutrición Hospitalaria*, 30/6 (2014), 1279–88

p. 56 Abrams, S. A. et al., 'A Combination of Prebiotic Short- and Long-Chain Inulin-Type Fructans Enhances Calcium Absorption and Bone Mineralization in Young Adolescents', *American Journal of Clinical Nutrition*, 82/2 (2005), 471–6

p. 58 Fang, N. et al., 'Inhibition of Growth and Induction of Apoptosis in Human Cancer Cell Lines by an Ethyl Acetate Fraction from Shiitake Mushrooms', *The Journal of Alternative and Complementary Medicine*, 12/2 (2006), 125–32 https://draxe.com/shiitake-mushrooms

WEEK FOUR

p. 62 Palkhivala, A., 'Glutathione: New Supplement on the Block', *MedicineNet.com* (30 July 2001) <http://www.medicinenet.com/script/main/art.asp?articlekey=50746>

p. 68 Thaiss, C. A. et al., 'Transkingdom Control of Microbiota Diurnal Oscillations Promotes Metabolic Homeostasis', *Cell*, 159/3 (2014), 514–29

p. 68 Anderson, G. & Maes, M., 'The Gut–Brain Axis: The Role of Melatonin in Linking Psychiatric, Inflammatory and Neurodegenerative Conditions', *Advances in Integrative Medicine*, 2/1 (2015), 31–7

p. 68 Mukherjee, S. & Maitra, S. K., 'Gut Melatonin in Vertebrates: Chronobiology and Physiology', *Frontiers in Endocrinology*, 6 (2015), 112

p. 69 http://www.webmd.com/diet/supplement-guide-magnesium#2-3

WEEK FIVE

p. 71 Korb, A., 'The Turkey-Tryptophan Myth', *Psychology Today* (21 November 2011) <https://www.psychologytoday.com/blog/prefrontal-nudity/201111/the-turkey-tryptophan-myth>

p. 71 http://nutritiondata.self.com/foods-02007900000000000000.html?maxCount=2

p. 71 http://nutritiondata.self.com/foods-01107900000000000000.html?maxCount=60

p. 71 Platkin, C., 'Sleep & Tryptophan', *Diet Detective* (19 November 2015) <http://www.dietdetective.com/sleep-tryptophan>

p. 73 Bested, A. C., Logan, A. C. & Selhub, E. M., 'Intestinal Microbiota, Probiotics and Mental Health: From Metchnikoff to Modern Advances: Part II – Convergence toward Clinical Trials', *Gut Pathogens*, 5/1 (2013), 4

p. 73 Lane, J. D. et al., 'Caffeine Effects on Cardiovascular and Neuroendocrine Responses to Acute Psychosocial Stress and Their Relationship to Level of Habitual Caffeine Consumption', *Psychosomatic Medicine*, 52/3 (1990), 320–36

p. 73 Maki, J., 'Berries Keep Your Brain Sharp', *Harvard Gazette* (26 April 2012) <http://news.harvard.edu/gazette/story/2012/04/berries-keep-your-brain-sharp>

p. 73 Mercola, J., 'Turmeric Compound Boosts Regeneration of Brain Stem Cells, and More', *Mercola.com* (13 October 2014) <http://articles.mercola.com/sites/articles/archive/2014/10/13/turmeric-curcumin.aspx>

p. 73 Kiecolt-Glaser J. K. et al., 'Daily Stressors, Past Depression, and Metabolic Responses To High-fat Meals: A Novel Path To Obesity', *Biological Psychiatry* (2015)

Stockists and Useful Resources

Lizearlewellbeing.com – Liz's own website to bookmark for updates and ongoing features on the latest on all aspects of gut health and gut-friendly recipes.

Kefirshop.co.uk – One of the UK's first and best suppliers of kefir and kombucha-making equipment and organic starter cultures, as well as original ginger beer 'plants'.

Red23.co.uk – An excellent superfood website selling fermented and cultured foods and drinks, including Body Ecology starter cultures, raw honeys and soil-based organisms (SBOs).

Evolutionorganics.co.uk – You'll find Dr Mercola's Kinetic Culture Starter Pack and other interesting and unusual gut-health supplements here.

Dr Alex Korb – A neuroscientist who consults and advises on links between microbes and depression. www.alexkorb.com https://alexkorbphd.wordpress.com/about/

A FEW FAVOURITES

Bio-Kult – makers of high-quality and award-winning probiotic capsules, including an advanced multi-strain formula containing fourteen live bacterial cultures proven to survive the high acidity of the stomach. www.bio-kult.com

Chuckling Goat – handmade live kefir from pasteurised or raw goat's milk, made using live kefir grains. www.chucklinggoat.co.uk

Dr Mercola – makers of the excellent Complete Probiotics supplement, containing ten strains of beneficial bacteria proven to survive stomach acids, plus additional prebiotics. www.drmercola. com

Jarr Kombucha – delicious genuine kombucha drinks packed in attractive dark glass bottles. www. jarrkombucha.com

Lewtress sparkling kombucha probiotic drinks – producing a wide range of flavours all containing live enzymes to aid digestion. One of the most delicious ways to drink kombucha. www.lewtress. co.uk

Sweet Cures – a good multi-strain probiotic supplement containing nine strains of beneficial bacteria plus a prebiotic. Sweet Cures also produce supplements specifically helpful for urinary tract infections, bladder health and cystitis. www.sweet-cures.com

Symprove – a liquid probiotic supplement made from the extract of germinated barley and containing four strains of live and active water-based bacteria, delivering approx. 10 billion colony-forming units (CFUs) per cupful. Useful as a first-off starter supplement. www.symprove.com

Vogel's Centaurium Centaury Drops – a useful digestive aid made from a tincture of bitter herbs, often taken to assist acid reflux.

VSL Powders – VSL#3 is an excellent probiotic powder containing a massive 450 billion live bacteria from eight different strains. I often recommend this as a kick-starter supplement taken with additional *L. rhamnosus*.

Glossary

Bacteria – the collective name for very small microorganisms. There are ten times more bacterial cells than human cells in the body. Some are beneficial and some are harmful. We need a good balance of beneficial bacteria for human health.

Cholesterol – a form of fat produced by the body and also obtained from some high-fat foods. There are two forms: LDL which is linked to heart disease, and HDL (known as the 'good' form of cholesterol) which can protect the heart.

Firmicutes – an anaerobic form of bacteria (does not use oxygen), these microbes make up the largest part of our gut microbiome and create energy from food. Firmicutes grow especially well on sugars and an excess is linked to obesity. Those who are overweight and obese have been found to have more Firmicutes in their gut.

Flora – meaning the plant life occurring in a specific region, flora can also refer to the overall bacteria, fungi and other microorganisms normally living in our gut.

FODMAP – an acronym that stands for Fermentable Oligosaccharides, Disaccharides, Monosaccharides And Polyols. These are a collection of sugars found in fruits, vegetables, dairy and wheat products. They can pass through the gut unchanged and are either fermented by bacteria in the colon or expelled with fluid, causing bloating, wind, abdominal pain and diarrhoea. Some find their digestive symptoms improve when following a FODMAP-free diet.

Gut – the overall term for the tube or tract that transfers food to our digestive organs, running from the mouth to the anus, with the oesophagus, stomach, small intestine and large intestine all part of this system. The human gastrointestinal tract is 9 metres (30 feet) long and filled with microbes that influence our hormones, enzymes and many other functions.

IBD – inflammatory bowel disease, a relatively rare condition which includes ulcerative colitis and Crohn's disease.

IBS – irritable bowel syndrome, a relatively common condition that causes stomach cramps, bloating, diarrhoea and/or constipation.

Inulin – a water-soluble dietary fibre found in plants, notably chicory. Inulin contains a mix of fructose polymer fibres that survive stomach acids to pass into the small intestine and feed beneficial bacteria living in the large intestine. High levels of inulin are linked to keeping us slim and healthy.

Lactoferrin – a cow's milk protein also found in human breast milk, tears and other body fluids such as bile. Lactoferrin regulates iron levels and helps prevent bad bacteria from causing infections. Linked to inhibiting lung cancer and improving acne.

Microbiome – the name given to the collective community of microorganisms that inhabit our gut.

Prebiotic – any specialised plant fibre that feeds our beneficial bacteria. High levels of prebiotics support a healthy gut.

Probiotic – live bacteria and yeasts with various health benefits, often referred to as our 'good' or 'friendly' bacteria.

Resistant starch – a type of dietary fibre found in many carbohydrates, including potatoes, grains and beans, especially when they have been cooked and cooled. Because it does not break down easily in the gut, it partly ferments, producing more beneficial bacteria and feeding others.

SBO – soil-based organisms or soil-based probiotics, these bacteria are different from other forms of probiotics as they don't live in the human gut but are found in the earth. SBOs are spores that come from the ground and research is under way into whether taking supplements could be beneficial for our health.

Symbiotic – also called a synbiotic, in this case it's a substance that contains both probiotics and prebiotics, ideal as the prebiotics are needed to feed the probiotics and help them flourish.

Acknowledgements

With special thanks to the Microbiome Medicine Summit for information from Dr Gerry Curatola and Ann Louise Gittleman, both speaking on the 2015 Microbiome Medicine Summit hosted by Raphael Kellman MD of the Kellman Center for Integrative and Functional Medicine (www.microbiomemedicinesummit.com) New York, New York. Also to Dr Josh Axe for his information about gut-healing herbs and probiotics. Thanks, too, to NatureDoc Lucinda Miller, Dr Ayesha Akbar, Sue Davis at Lifehouse Spa, Dr Rangan Chatterjee, Elena Voyce PhD and Barry Smith at Symprove.

This has been such a wonderfully inspiring book to write. From my initial concept to its creative fruition, I am so grateful to the incredibly talented team of people who turned my dream into reality on these pages. Firstly, my literary agent Rosemary Sandberg and publishing director Amanda Harris, and all at Orion Spring, notably Olivia Morris whose careful eye has guided every page. I'm grateful to Katy Sunnassee for her research and drafting, to copy-editor Sue Phillpott, dietician Fiona Hunter and recipe developer Heather Whinney.

On the creative side, I'd like to thank Dan Jones for his wonderful photography, assisted by Sophie Fox and Sam Folan, also Patrick Drummond for his farm photography and Tamzin Ferdinando for her fabulous styling. Also thanks to Natalie Thomson for her delicious food styling, assisted by Iona Blackshaw and Laura Urschel, all under the watchful eye of creative director Helen Ewing. I am always grateful to make-up artist Kerry September and hair stylist Jon Malone, as well as to Lily Earle for wardrobe styling. Thanks are also due to my commercial and brand director Polly Beard and to my talented team at the Liz Earle Wellbeing Studios. I am truly thrilled that this book looks as beautiful as its important and life-changing contents surely merit. Thank you.

Credits:

Cover and pages 2, 63: sweater, Valentino
Page 31, 95: blouse, Yvonne Damant
Page 43, 48: dressing gown, Christian Dior
Page 46, 83, 105, 111, 163: sweater, Max Mara
Page 55, 60: clothing, Jaeger
Page 60: sportswear, Sweaty Betty
Page 67: sweater, ME+EM
Page 75: top, Feather and Bone

Page 121: shirt, Ralph Lauren; apron The Linen Works
Page 135: dress, Goat
Page 199: dress, Valentino
Page 225: sweater, Max Mara; apron Liz's own
Page 231: tops, vintage
Page 237: sweater, Brora

Jewellery – Liz Earle Fair and Fine Botany Collections, available from Cred.com
With special thanks to The White Company for kitchen props

OVEN TEMPERATURE GUIDE

	Elec °C	Elec °F	Elec °C (Fan)	Gas mark
Very cool	110	225	90	¼
	120	250	100	½
Cool	140	275	120	1
	150	300	130	2
Moderate	160	325	140	3
	170	350	160	4
Moderately hot	190	375	170	5
	200	400	180	6
Hot	220	425	200	7
	230	450	210	8
Very hot	240	475	220	9

WEIGHT MEASUREMENTS

Metric	Imperial
10g	½ oz
20g	¾ oz
25g	1 oz
40g	1½ oz
50g	2 oz
60g	2½ oz
75g	3 oz
110g	4 oz
125g	4½ oz
150g	5 oz
175g	6 oz
200g	7 oz
225g	8 oz
250g	9 oz
275g	10 oz
350g	12 oz
450g	1 lb
700g	1½ lb
900g	2 lb

LIQUID MEASUREMENTS (under 1 litre)

Metric	Imperial	Australian/US
25ml	1 fl oz	
60ml	2 fl oz	¼ cup
75ml	3 fl oz	
100ml	3½ fl oz	
120ml	4 fl oz	½ cup
150ml	5 fl oz	
180ml	6 fl oz	¾ cup
200ml	7 fl oz	
250ml	9 fl oz	1 cup
300ml	10½ fl oz	1¼ cups
350ml	12½ fl oz	1½ cups
400ml	14 fl oz	1¾ cups
450ml	16 fl oz	2 cups
600ml	1 pint	2½ cups
750ml	1¼ pints	3 cups
900ml	1½ pints	3½ cups

LIQUID MEASUREMENTS (over 1 litre)

Metric	Imperial	Australian/US
1 litre	1¾ pints	1 quart or 4 cups
1.2 litres	2 pints	
1.4 litres	2½ pints	
1.5 litres	2¾ pints	
1.7 litres	3 pints	
2 litres	3½ pints	

General Index

diabetes 16, 76, 78
  type 2 17
diarrhoea 15, 16, 29, 51, 52,
    53, 64, 77, 93
diets, special 10, 12, 16, 23,
    40, 42, 43, 49, 56, 61, 70,
    73, 76, 78, 81, 86
digestion, easing 74, 92
digestivejuices 10
digestive system 11–13, 15, *also*
    see gut
dizziness 30
DNA 10
Drake, Karen Sinclair 48
duodenum 11
dysbiosis 13, *57*, 68, 73

E. coli 29, 30
eating: disorders 39, 40
  mindfully *74*, 79, 94
eczema 12, 92
enzymes 8, 10, 14, 33, *57*, 81,
    85, 87
EPA 86
exercise, importance of 13, 64–5,
    94

facial massage 68
faeces, *see* stools
fasting 10, 23, 34
fatigue 14, 16, 17, 27, 44, 58,
    62
fats 11, 41, 73
fennel *57*, 91, 93
fermented food 59, 81–6, 93,
    94
fibre 12, 77, 79
firmicutes 16, 23
fish, oily 41, 86
flatulence 52, *see also* gas
flax seed 41–2, 86
folic acid 16
FODMAP foods 24, 42, *57*
folate-rich foods 62
food 10, 24–5, 37
fruit 38, 42, 55–6, 59, 76, 77,
    79, 82, 85, 90, *see also*
  avocado, cranberries dried 24,

76

gall bladder 11
garlic 28, 33, 42, *57*, 82
gas (tapped wind) 13, 15, 16,
    46, *57*, *see also* flatulence
gastritis 63
gastroenteritis 29, 52
gastrointestinal (GI) 13, 16, 40,
    90
  tract 9, 10, 11, *11*, 26, 33,
    34, 36, 37, 46, 64, 77, 94
ginger *73*, 84
ginger ale 84
glucose 11, 12, 24, 41, 68
glutathione 62
gluten 14, 15, 16, 17, 18, 24,
    28, 34
grains 15, 24, 38, 61, 76, 77,
    79, 86, 90, 93
grapefruit seed extract 29–30
gut, 10–15, 15–19, 19, 23, 25,
    33, 36, 37, 38, 39, 40,
    40–1, 62, 66, 71, *see also*
  antioxidant, bacteria, Bentonite,
    detoxification, microbiome,
    oral hygiene, probiotics,
    Psyllium, skin and skin health
    47–8
  good gut checklist 34, 49, 59,
    69, 79, 94
  gut health 70–9, 86
  influence on emotions 70–3
  leaky 18, *18*, 2

headaches 16, 42, 81
heart disease 13, 16, 62, *77*
heartburn 44, 63, 89
herbal detoxifiers 28, 34
herbs 28, 34, 49, 56, 64, 78,
    82, 91–3
honey 24, 47, 58, 85
hormones 19, 39, 40, 41, 52,
    68, 73, 76
hypochlorhydria 44

ileum 11
immune system 8, 13, 16, 17,

    18, 19, 37, 39, 40, 48, 51,
    52, 53, 58, 59, 62, 64,
    90, 93
indigestion 14, 30, 74, 78, 92
infections, fighting 30
infertility 24
inflammation 14, 73
inflammatory bowel disease (IBD)
    15, 17, 51
insulin 29, 41, 76, 78
intestines 9, 13, 14, 15, 16, 17,
    41, 51, 53, 64, 65, 71, 86
  small 10, 11, 14, 15, 26–8,
    34, 53, 87
  large 11, 12, *12*, 30, 53,
    54, 55, 77, 87, 89
iron 16
irritable bowl syndrome (IBS) 15,
    16, 17, 22, 40, 42, 51,
    78, 90

jejunum 11

kefir 85
Kimchi 82
Kombucha 25, 34, 46, 59, 79,
    82, 84, 92, 94
Korb, Alex 71
Kvass 25, 34, 80, 82

lactoferrin 47, 49
lentils 38, 62, *77*
liquorice: and peppermint tea 91
  root 63, 69
lupus 16, 17
lymphatic system 13

magnesium 26, 33, 69, 86, 94
  bath 61
meditation 94
mental health 17
microbes 8, 9, 10, 11, 12, 13,
    14, 16, 17, 19, 23, 29, 33,
    37, 38, 40, 41, 42, 47,
    48, 52, 54, 55, 56, 58,
    68, 72, *see also* firmicutes,
    gut, skin, weight gain
microbiome 8–9, 9, 10, 13, 16,

17, 22, 24, 25, 36–49, 38, 40, 43, 47, 52, 53, 68, 78, see also
detoxification, oral hygiene tips for health 43–4
microflora 22, 51
migraines 59, 81
milk 28, 33, 47, 48, 51, 53, 56, 59, 71, 76, 85, 93
from the breast 37–8
Miller, Lucinda 44
minerals 11
mint 43, 92, 93
MS 16, 17
mushrooms, medicinal 58–9, 66

nausea 16, 27,
nettle tea 92
neuro-immuno-cutaneous-endocrine (NICE) network 19
nightshade foods 42
non-coeliac gluten sensitivity (NCGS) 16, 24
nuts 17, 41, 61, 62, 73, 74, 76, 78, 90

obesity 13, 16, 23, 37, 38, 40, 76, 82, see also weight gain

oesophagus 10, 28
older age 40–2
olive leaf extract 30
Omega-3s 41, 48, 73, 86
oral hygiene 43–4, 49
oregano oil 29, 34
organic food 24, 43, 55–6, 59, 66, 71, 85, 93

pain 13, 14, 15, 16, 52, 73,
pancreas 11
panic attacks, alleviating 76
Parkinson's disease 17, 41
pathogens 52
peppermint, see liquorice
pilates 65
plaque, importance of 43
pollen 17, 58
poultry 69, 71, 76

prebiotics 28, 40, 41, 42, 54, 56–7, 58, 78, 80
probiotics 13, 19, 22, 25, 30, 40–1, 50, 51, 52, 53, 54–5, 56, 58, 59, 60, 74, 78, 80, 82, 84, 85, 94
face mask 47
protein 11, 15, 16, 33, 37, 38, 44, 49, 58, 63, 71, 76, 90
psoriasis 17
Psyllium Cleanse, the 28, 34, 94
pulses 56, 77, 79, 93
pumpkin seed 28, 33, 61

reflexology, foot 68
rheumatoid arthritis 16

sauerkraut 74, 80, 81, 82, 93, 94
schizophrenia 17, 39
seed, easing digestion of 90
selenium-rich foods 62
serotonin 70
short-chain fatty acids (SCFA) 12
skin 9, 10, 14, 15, 16, 19, 23, 30, 37, 39, 42, 47–8, 61, 66, 81
sleep, 27, 58, 66, 68
Slippery elm 64
small intestinal bowel overgrowth (SIBO) 15, 29
smoking 44
sourdough 24, 82, 86
spirulina 63, 66, 71
starches, resistant to digestion 78
stomach 10, 15
acid 44–6, 49
stools (faeces) 13, 14, 15, 17, 37, 77, 89, 93
stress 13, 39, 40, 44, 52, 64, 73, 74, 76, 94, see also
anxiety coping with 52, 56, 58, 61, 68, 69, 73, 74, 87
sugar 11, 12, 24, 40, 41, 76, see also blood sugar, sweeteners
sugars, calorific 24

sushi 78
sweeteners, artificial 24
symbiotics 40

teenagers 39, 40, 41
thrush, vaginal 30, 52
triphala 93
tryptophan-rich foods 71
turmeric 73

ulcers 28, 63
urinary tract infections 29

vagus nerve 72
vegetables 33, 38, 41, 40, 42, 49, 56, 57, 62, 76, 77, 79, see also
beetroot, broccoli, potatoes
grow your own 55–6
juice 94
vitamins 8, 11
B 82; B1 44; B6 44;
B12 11, 16, 82; C 62, 78, 82
D 61; E 47, 62; K2 61
vomiting 16

water, drinking levels 78, 94
weight 15, 16, 68
wormwood 30, 34
worms 33

yoga 65, 68, 87–9, 93

zinc 33, 44, 86

Recipe Index

About Liz

Liz Earle MBE is one of Britain's most respected and trusted authorities on wellbeing. The award-winning author of over 30 best-selling books on nutrition, diet, beauty and natural healthcare, she co-founded the eponymous global beauty brand Liz Earle Beauty Co. in 1995, before moving back to writing and broadcasting, now publishing the leading quarterly magazine *Liz Earle Wellbeing*.

An expert in feel-good food and eating well to look good, her straightforward, balanced and well-researched approach has earned her a place as a trusted visionary in the world of wellbeing. With a passion for demystifying science and sharing wellness wisdom, Liz's measured voice of reason has a deservedly large and loyal following in print, on digital, on TV and online.

Travelling the globe for research, Liz comes home to roost on an organic farm in the UK's West Country with her husband and five children.

Sign up to Liz's free *Wellbeing* newsletter with new gut-friendly recipes and advice: www.lizearlewellbeing.com

FOLLOW LIZ

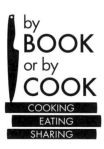

Facebook: Liz Earle Wellbeing

Instagram: @LizEarleWellbeing

YouTube: Liz Earle Wellbeing

Pinterest: Liz Earle Wellbeing

Twitter: @LizEarleWb

Snapchat: LizEarleWb

Also by Liz Earle

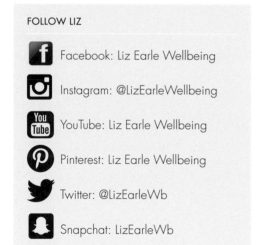

For more delicious recipes, features, videos and exclusives from Orion's cookery writers, and to sign up for our 'Recipe of the Week' email visit **bybookorbycook.co.uk**

Follow Orion

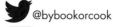 @bybookorcook

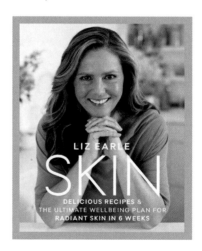 @bybookorbycook

Find us

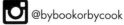 facebook.com/bybookorbycook